Hand Recovery after Stroke
Exercises and Results Measurements

Hand Recovery after Stroke
Exercises and Results Measurements

Johannes G. Smits, Ph.D.
Associate Professor, Electrical and Computer Engineering, Boston University, Boston

Else C. Smits-Boone
Artist, Poet

Foreword by Catherine A. Trombly Sc.D., OTR/L, FAOTA
Professor of Occupational Therapy, Sargent College of Health and
Rehabilitation Sciences, Boston University, Boston

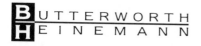

Boston Oxford Auckland Johannesburg Melbourne New Delhi

Every effort has been made to ensure that the drug dosage schedules within this text are accurate and conform to standards accepted at time of publication. However, as treatment recommendations vary in light of continuing research and clinical experience, the reader is advised to verify drug dosage schedules herein with information found on product information sheets. This is especially true in cases of new or infrequently used drugs.

♾ Recognizing the importance of preserving what has been written, Butterworth–Heinemann prints its books on acid-free paper whenever possible.

 Butterworth–Heinemann supports the efforts of American Forests and the Global ReLeaf program in its campaign for the betterment of trees, forests, and our environment.

Library of Congress Cataloging-in-Publication Data
Smits, Johannes Gerardus, 1944-
    Hand recovery after stroke : exercise and results measurements/Johannes G. Smits,
Else Smits-Boone.
      p. cm.
    Includes index.
    ISBN 0-7506-7272-2 (alk. paper)
      1. Cerebrovascular disease--Exercise therapy. 2. Cerebrovascular
disease--Patients--Rehabilitation. 3. Hand--Diseases--Exercise therapy. I. Smits-Boone,
Else. II. Title

RC388.5 .S64 2000
616.8'106515--dc21   00-030408

British Library Cataloguing-in-Publication Data
A catalogue record for this book is available from the British Library.

The publisher offers special discounts on bulk orders of this book.
For information, please contact:
Manager of Special Sales
Butterworth–Heinemann
225 Wildwood Avenue
Woburn, MA 01801-2041
Tel: 781-904-2500
Fax: 781-904-2640

For information on all Butterworth–Heinemann publications available,
contact our World Wide Web home page at: http://www.bh.com

10 9 8 7 6 5 4 3 2 1

Printed in the United States of America

Contents

You go to the hospital,
They explain everything,
You do not hear.
They calm you down with words,
You do not understand.
No, you cannot go with him,
He is not doing so well; we do not understand him.
I do.
It is the language of survival.
You go home, frightened,
He is paralyzed.
You call the family,
They do not understand.
Days later you understand he has had
A severe stroke.
So you start fighting.

—Else

Foreword

In the past, no books were available to patients interested in continuing rehabilitation of hand function after their formal rehabilitation ended. Dr. Johannes Smits, a stroke survivor, devised the exercises in this book for himself and, after noting continued recovery well past the time his recovery was expected to end, wrote this book to guide and inspire others. In *Hand Recovery after Stroke: Exercises and Results Measurements*, he shares his observations and feelings about stroke recovery "from the inside out"—something therapists who have not experienced a stroke cannot do. Johannes, together with his co-author and wife, Else Smits-Boone, encourages all stroke survivors on their path to recovery, providing useful examples for all readers to follow.

Recovering from a stroke is different for everyone. Some people regain full use of their affected arm and hand while others regain only rudimentary movement. This book's message is that with practice, improvement in hand function can happen. In conveying this message, the book provides places for readers to record their daily scores in order to track their own progress. This tracking is part of a special feature Dr. Smits has developed to help readers estimate their recovery time for particular hand functions and decide when to switch from an active therapy program to a maintenance mode of therapy. These features also help readers recognize that although much work is required to progress, small changes may eventually result in useful movement.

Although this book was written to fill a pragmatic need, it is not without scientific basis. It has long been known that millions of repetitions are required to develop any motor skill. This is especially true of the development of voluntary movement from the reflex-based movement that occurs after stroke.[1] Research using advanced imaging techniques that record brain activity in primates and humans indicates that the brain tissue reorganizes as movements are relearned after a stroke.[2-3] The speed and smoothness of movement improve with practice.[4] This need for practice and repetition is evident in babies as they develop hand movement: they start by moving in gross, general patterns of movement; bit by bit they "practice" until their movements become more refined. The day a baby uses a single finger to precisely push the "ON" button on the TV remote, she has mastered a new skill that has taken countless hours of practice to accomplish.

The exercises in this manual utilize common objects to accomplish real-life goals. These common objects help the reader organize movement after stroke better than pure exercise does.[5-6] It should comfort readers that Dr. Smits engages in these same exercises every day himself. You may not be able to accomplish as much as he does, but you should see some improvement in the movements that you choose to practice. Good luck and best wishes as you strive to put both hands back to work in your daily life!

Catherine A. Trombly, Sc.D., OTR/L

References

1. Kottke, F.J. (1980). From reflex to skill: The training of coordination. *Archives of Physical Medicine and Rehabilitation, 61,* 551-561.

2. Nudo, R.J., Wise, B.M., SiFuentes, F., & Milliken, G.W. (1996). Neural substrates for the effects of rehabilitative training on motor recovery after ischemic infarct. *Science, 272,* 1791-1794.

3. Karni, A., Meyer, G., Jezzard, P., Adams, M.M., Turner, R., & Ungerleider, L.G. (1995). Functional MRI evidence for adult motor cortex plasticity during motor skill learning. *Nature, 377,* 155-158.

4. Trombly, C.A. (1993). Observations of improvement of reaching in five subjects with left hemiparesis. *Journal of Neurology, Neurosurgery, and Psychiatry, 56,* 40-45.

5. Wu, C-y, Trombly, C.A., Lin, K-c, & Tickle-Degnen, L. (1998). Effects of object affordances on reaching performance in persons with and without cerebrovascular accident. *American Journal of Occupational Therapy, 52,* 447-456.

6. Trombly, C.A., & Wu, C-y. (In press). The effect of rehabilitation tasks on the organization of movement post stroke. *American Journal of Occupational Therapy.*

Acknowledgments

We would like to thank all those who have helped us when Johannes was recovering from his stroke. Special thanks go to Wendy Burton, Amy Markey, Melissa Portnoy, and Nancy Milch, all therapists at the Braintree Rehabilitation Hospital in Braintree, Massachusetts. We would also like to thank Professor Cathy A. Trombly of the Boston University Sargent College, School for Physical Medicine and Rehabilitation, Department of Occupational Therapy, who suggested that we write this book. Also thanks to Dr. Serge H. Roy of the Neuromuscular Research Center in the College of Engineering's Biomedical Engineering Department. We would also like to thank Professor Dr. Lucia M. Vaina of the Department of Biomedical Engineering at Boston University for her invaluable help with early vision problems.

We would also like to thank our brother/brother-in-law Leo Smits for jumping on a plane and making a weekend round-trip transatlantic flight to lend his help and comfort in the first weekend following Johannes' stroke. We would also like to thank Yvonne Smits-Ruijsink, our sister-in-law, who is a physical therapist with her own practice in The Hague in the Netherlands, for coming over a few weeks later and for helping Johannes to move his hand again. We would also like to thank Johannes' parents for making daily and weekly calls to support us with words of wisdom, sympathy, and consolation.

We would also like to thank the Trustees of Boston University for allowing us to write this book using its computer systems.

Last but not least we would like to thank our good neighbors, Dr. Jane Murphy Gaughan and Dr. Gerry Gaughan, for their support and help, and for evolving from good neighbors into dear friends.

Johannes Smits, Else Smits-Boone

Preface: For Whom This Book Was Written

Every year, around 500,000 Americans—or about one out of every 500 people—suffer a stroke, a form of brain damage caused by interruption of the blood supply to a part of the brain. Of these 500,000, around 150,000 die. The damaged part of the brain may be as small as a pea or as large as the patient's fist. Stroke survivors become paralyzed on one or two sides, and may suffer partial or complete blindness. If survivors can see, they may not be able to read. Survivors may also be oversensitive to light and sound, lose their hearing or their sense of touch on the side that is paralyzed, and may not feel the difference between hot and cold. Survivors may also be disoriented and unable to remember their name, address, phone number, the alphabet, the current date or year, or how to count. When the stroke occurs on the left side, the right side is paralyzed, and, because the language center is on the left side of the brain, survivors may not be able to speak. Many stroke survivors have permanent damage but are so clever at hiding their deficiencies that only a trained physician, therapist, or another stroke survivor who is equally adept at hiding a stroke deficiency will notice. At any rate, suffering a stroke is one of the most severe traumas a person can survive, on par with a heart attack or cancer.

Strokes can happen to people of any age, including children as young as two years old who suffer from a genetic defect of one of the arteries feeding the brain. Many stroke survivors are relatively young and would otherwise have many years of life ahead of them. Some are adults who suffer an injury to one of the arteries—possibly sports-related or owing to a sudden head motion. Other stroke survivors have clogged arteries, or the inner lining of one of their arteries may have delaminated from the outer wall. Some people who suffer a stroke have various risk factors, including diabetes and high blood pressure, while other people, including the author of this book, have no known risk factors for stroke at all.

The author of this book is a healthy, 51-year-old male scientist, physicist, engineer, and university professor who maintained a vigorous lifestyle until one day while working in his lab he noticed that he was partially blind and had lost sensation in his left hand. A few hours later, he suffered a massive stroke for reasons that are not yet resolved and that may never be. After weeks of hospital treatment and several months of rehabilitation, he was discharged from the hospital. He could not walk very well; he had no sensation in his left side; he could not use his left hand. He had found a way to bend his fingers, but could not straighten them after bending. He could not pick up objects; he could not hold a glass of water, or a fork, spoon, or knife. He had lost a great deal of control over the muscles of his throat so that he often choked on his food and bit his tongue even when speaking. He did not even remember the alphabet completely. When therapy could no longer help him recover, he decided to use his scientific problem-solving approach to tackle his own recovery. He went to libraries and bookstores to research rehabilitation exercises that he could do at home, but found none. He thus decided to write the book that he would have bought if it had existed.

This book is a report of the author's own recovery process, as well as a complete and detailed description of the exercises he designed for himself and performed on a daily basis. It has been written so that others who are similarly affected by a stroke can perform the exercises and improve their health as well as the author has been able to. It has been written for the many people who suffer a stroke and find themselves in a hospital bed or wheelchair, unable to work and dependent on family members, friends, or good neighbors for the continuation of their lives. These stroke patients have only one burning desire: to get back to normal as fast as they can.

None of the exercises in this book involves the use of medications other than those medications your doctor already prescribes. To use this book you don't need any particular education in occupational therapy, or in anything else. This book presumes that you can read normal English (put on your glasses if necessary!), and that you are able to write a number with one hand. It is also presumed that you can draw a cross with one hand. While that presumption may be unrealistic for those of you whose dominant hand has been paralyzed and who thus only have your non-dominant hand to work with, you may still be able to do these tasks. If you are not able to record a number or draw a cross, a family member or good friend may be able to do so. You will also have to take measurements of the time it takes to perform certain tasks, and you will have to convert those measurements into minutes and seconds from the stopwatch's seconds-only reading. Use a calculator if you want.

Although it is presumed that you can do these things, it is not strictly necessary. What is necessary is that you **DO** the exercises. Don't worry about the background knowledge you may not have. If you can draw a line from one point to another using a pencil and a ruler, if you can measure the length of a line with the ruler, you are set to go. The most important thing is that you **DO** the exercises.

Since the majority of stroke patients get in-patient and outpatient rehabilitation, this book has also been written for therapists. The ideal situation is for the stroke patient and therapist to go over these exercises together, with the therapist teaching the patient how to perform the exercises, measure his or her performance, and record and plot that performance in the graphs in this book. The best time for such training is when the stroke patient visits on an outpatient basis, several times a week for three to four months. We suggest the therapist teach the patient a new exercise every day, and give this book to the patient for home exercises.

It is a testimony to the resilience and adaptability of the human species that a majority of stroke survivors find a way in which they either regain some, most, or all of their faculties, or find a way of living in which they compensate for their defects. The implied question that forms the title of this preface can now be answered: This book has been written for all stroke survivors and their therapists.

One final note: the "I" referred to in this book is Johannes. (Many of the observations of Johannes's recovery progress, or lack thereof, were made by Else.)

1

Ten Reasons to Do the Exercises in This Book

There are a number of very good reasons why you should do the exercises in this book. These reasons include:

1. Exercise will help you gradually return your affected limb to an approximately normal state.
2. Exercise gives you the feeling that you are back in control of your life.
3. Exercise actually produces a positive feeling—a sort of high—and it dramatically improves your sense of well being. Although the cause is not yet entirely understood, exercise affects the levels of the brain's neurotransmitters, including adrenaline. Researchers have found that adrenogenic drugs (drugs that stimulate the formation of adrenaline), when combined with exercise, improve recovery from brain damage in monkeys.
4. Exercise improves the blood circulation in the affected limb.
5. Exercise reduces the stiffening of the muscle tissue in the affected limb.
6. Exercise gives you an important record of your improvement. Many people, when they hear that you have had a stroke, will tell you how good you look and how much better you appear to be doing than the last time they saw you. In the meantime, however, you may notice no progress whatsoever and become depressed. In fact, depression is so common that the Agency for Health Care Policy Research's *Guidelines for the Treatment of Stroke Patients* explicitly instructs hospital staffs to assume that stroke patients are or will become depressed, given that the illness has such traumatic effects. However, if you exercise and record your performance every day, you will notice slow improvements, and your depression may dissipate.
7. The disability insurance company that is supposed to help you through this difficult time—if you have this coverage—may do everything they can to avoid having to pay your benefits. (My insurance company did not want to pay disability benefits and used all the terms in the contract to avoid having to pay.) It is smart to keep a record of your improvements (or lack thereof) in case you need it.

8. If you don't exercise, the muscles that have atrophied somewhat due to the paralysis will atrophy even further, making it more difficult to regain normal use of your affected limb.

9. My own personal research has indicated that exercises lead to improvements (in my case, around 0.1 to 1 percent per day, depending on the exercise). The same research has revealed that the deterioration caused by not exercising is quite severe (in my case, around 5 percent per day). Although I have no concrete proof, I feel that this deterioration is mainly due to muscle stiffening, not atrophy. After a period of not exercising, the limb's old condition is not immediately recovered. It may take days to recover the loss of a week of not exercising. If you don't exercise for a day, you don't just lose the progress of that day's exercise. Due to muscle stiffening, you effectively lose almost ten days worth of exercise. You need around three days of exercise to recover those ten days and to return your body to its performance level of the day before you skipped the exercise. In all, one day of not exercising sets you back around two weeks. The moral of this story: Do your exercises! (The numbers quoted here are based on my experience; your stroke may be more or less severe.)

10. Pain in the affected limb can be quite severe—even unbearable. The pain may be caused by poor blood circulation, muscle atrophy, or coagulation of muscle tissue. Although a physician can prescribe medication to treat this pain, exercise can also help relieve it. Pain generally disappeared in my arm after a normal daily exercise routine, and stayed away the rest of the day. The pain returned two or three days later if I did not exercise. The disappearance of the pain may have been caused by better oxygenation of the arm and hand, or by the removal of muscle-stiffening proteins. Whatever the reason, the removal of unbearable pain was an unintended but welcome side effect of the exercises.

2

What the Experts Say about Stroke Recovery

It is widely believed that hemiplegic stroke survivors can be rehabilitated somewhat, but most research indicates that rehabilitation occurs primarily in the first three to six months following the stroke. Health insurance companies take this belief into consideration when a patient requests more occupational or physical therapy. These insurance companies sometimes reject requests for rehabilitation past the three- to six-month mark based on the belief that more therapy will not be helpful. This chapter will present a brief review of stroke rehabilitation based on a number of research papers from rehabilitation literature.

Researchers have found differences in the rehabilitation of the upper extremity with respect to the lower extremity; this is due to the fact that the upper extremity requires more fine motor control than the lower extremity.[1] Meanwhile, it is an accepted practice to evaluate stroke patients after three months of rehabilitation and again after six months. Often, no significant difference in Activities of Daily Living (ADL) function can be found.[2] Depending on the severity of the stroke, a prognosis can be given about the patient's recovery at this time. Best ADL function is reached within five weeks in patients with initially mild disability, in nine weeks in patients with initially moderate disability, and in sixteen to seventeen weeks in patients with very severe disability.[2] However, return of neurological, motor, and sensory functions should not be expected after five months in patients with a severe stroke.[2]

Recovery curves can be used to predict the outcome of continued rehabilitation.[3] Researchers use descriptive analysis (such as, "patient does/does not perform an action") rather than quantitative analysis to determine the value of one therapy over another.[4-5] Usually, statistical methods with large numbers of patients are needed to assess the quality of rehabilitation.[6] However, the process underlying recovery from stroke, its time course, and the importance of therapeutic interventions in the promotion of recovery are not clear.[7]

To some extent, the brain can repair itself by assigning undamaged parts to the functions lost in the damaged part.[6] This has been studied using primates who received a lesion to the brain.[8] When highly stereotyped, repetitive training of the same movement is performed, the relearning of tasks is superior to conventional physiotherapy in which less emphasis is placed on repetitive exercising.[8]

Nevertheless, regaining complete control over the hand, including independent control over the digits, is rare, at least in humans.[9]

Meanwhile, muscles that operate together in a task appear to be represented together in the cortex,[10] indicating that the brain learns to perform tasks, rather than the individual use of muscles. During the recovery process, the patient may experience super-sensitivity because undamaged neurons in the presence of the damaged neurons may also become abnormal.[11]

This is what research papers tell us about stroke rehabilitation. However, the basic tenet of this workbook is that the statements made in the existing literature are not completely correct. On the contrary, I have discovered that recovery goes on nearly as long as the patient keeps on performing exercises. I have written a paper on my findings, which was accepted in the *Journal of Neurovascular Disease* and is printed in its entirety as Appendix II of this book.

References

1. Duncan, P.W., Goldstein, L.B., Horner, R.D., Landsman, P.B., Samsa, G.P., & Matchar, D.B. (1994). Similar motor recovery of upper and lower extremities after stroke. *Stroke, 25(6),* 1181–1188.

2. Jorgensen, H.S., Nakayama, H., Raaschou, H.O., Vive-Larsen, J., Stoier, M., & Olsen, T.S. (1955). Outcome and time course of recovery in stroke, part I: Outcome. The Copenhagen stroke study. *Arch. Phys. Med Rehabil, 76,* 399–405.

3. Partridge, C.J., & Edwards, S. (1988). Recovery curves as basis for evaluation. *Physiotherapy, 74(3),* 141–143.

4. Partridge, C.J. (1992). Describing patterns of recovery as a basis for evaluating progress. *International Journal on Technology Assessment in Health Care, 8(1),* 55–61.

5. Parker, V.M., Wade, T.D., & Langton Hewer, R. (1986). Loss of arm function after stroke, measurement frequency and recovery. *Int. Rehabil.Med, 8,* 69–73.

6. Duncan, P.W., Goldstein, L.B., Matchar, D., Divine, G.W., & Feussner J. (1992). Measurement of motor recovery after stroke. *Stroke, 23(8),* 1084–1089.

7. Dombovy, M.L., & Bach-y-Rita, P. (1988). Clinical observations on recovery from stroke. *Advances in Neurology, 47,* Functional recovery in neurological Disease. New York: Raven Press.

8. Freund, H.J. (1996). Remapping the brain. *Science, 272,* 1754.

9. Nudo, R.J., Wise, B.M., SiFuentes, F., Milliken, G.W. (1996). Neural substrates for the effects of rehabilitative training on motor recovery after ischemic infarct. *Science, 272,* 1791–1794.

10. Nudo, R.J., Milliken, G.W., Jenkins, W.M., & Merzenich, M.M. (1966) Use dependent alterations of movement representations in primary motor cortex on adult squirrel monkeys. *J. NeuroScience, 16(2),* 785–809.

11. Brunnstrom, S. (1970). *Movement therapy in hemiplegia.* New York: Harper & Row.

How a Recovery Process Can Be Described

Almost all naturally developing processes are smooth functions of time, changing gradually, slowly or quickly, but without sudden changes in the process. The amount a child grows each day is so small that it doesn't make sense to measure the growth more than once a month. However, if we did measure this growth with sufficient accuracy, we would see changes taking place on a daily basis. Other processes go faster; for example, kittens become adult cats in roughly one year, and although we don't measure their growth every day, we would see changes if we did take such measurements.

So what do growth cycles of children and kittens have to do with stroke survivors? If you have had a stroke, you may notice that you are not recovering as fast as you had hoped you would. You may feel that you are not recovering at all, that you are stuck, or that you have "plateaued," as therapists call it. It is important to remember, however, that recovery from a stroke is one such barely noticeable, slow process. The growth of a city, the development of an ant colony, the production of cells in a developing fetus—these are all examples of well studied and analyzed cases. So, too, can the recovery from a stroke be measured, plotted, and analyzed.

The recovery of stroke patients takes place in what is called an "exponential decay process." This means that the performance of stroke patients, as measured in the amount of time it takes them to finish a certain task, follows the same rules and patterns as many other well-known processes. In this book it is assumed that my recovery—and, in turn, your own recovery—is in no way unusual. You may find that your recovery process is different from mine, or it may be similar in certain exercises and vastly different in others. In any case, all stroke survivors follow the exponential decay process.

To understand how the recovery process develops, we will discuss a familiar process that behaves identically to the stroke recovery process. Because the basic concepts of the process are important, we will cover them in great detail.

As an example, let's perform an experiment: Consider the water level in a leaking bucket. In the beginning, the bucket is filled to a level of 10 inches. Now, assume that there is a small leak at the bottom of the bucket. If we take a ruler and measure the height of the water level every 10 minutes and write down that measurement, we will get a table similar to Table 3–1.

Table 3–1   Water Level as Function of Time

Time (in minutes)	Height (in inches)
0 (start)	10
10	5
20	2.5
30	1.25
40	0.625
50	0.3125
60	0.15625
70	0.078125
80	0.0390625
90	0.01953125

A plot of the height of the water level is shown in Figure 3–1. The time is marked on the horizontal line; as you see, there is a mark for each of the times mentioned from the start (at time zero) until the end (at 90 minutes). At each of these points, a small diamond figure marks the height of the water level in the bucket. You can see how high the water level is at each of the diamonds by looking at the vertical line and reading its corresponding value. Straight lines connect the points. Thus, when you wish to read a level somewhere between two measured values—for instance, when you want to know the water's height after 26 minutes—you will need to look at the nearest measurements—in this case, those performed at 20 and 30 minutes, respectively. This means that, in our example, at 26 minutes, the water level is between the level indicated at the 20- and 30-minute mark. Therefore, the level at 26 minutes is somewhere between 2 1/2 and 1 1/4 inches.

If you want a more accurate reading of the water level at 26 minutes, mark a cross where 26 minutes would fall on the horizontal line. Then, draw a vertical line through that cross until it intersects with the straight line that connects the two diamonds at 2 1/2 and 1 1/4 inches. Mark that intersection with a circle. Now draw a straight horizontal line through that circle until it intersects the vertical line. Mark that intersection with another cross. Notice that the height is slightly less than 2 inches, and that although there is no tick mark on the vertical height line for that point, you can estimate the height quite accurately. Note that a smooth line has also been drawn in the graph, represented by the dotted line. This line represents the height if continuous measurements were taken every second instead of every 10 minutes.

You may notice a peculiarity in this process: after 10 minutes, the water level is just half the level at the start, while after 10 more minutes, the level is again half of what it was at the start of the second 10-minute period. This rate remains constant throughout the process.

Now, imagine that you have a second bucket that is the same as the first bucket, and that you also fill it with water to the same height. However, in this example the hole through which the water leaks is twice as big. Again, measurements are made every 10 minutes, and are plotted on the same graph (Figure 3–1). In this example, the points are indicated by small plus signs (+) to distinguish them from the first set of measurements (which was marked by small diamonds). These measurements are represented by a smooth curve, as in the previous example, and are represented by the dotted line on the graph. For this example as in the last, imagine that this dotted line represents the height if continuous measurements were taken every second instead of every 10 minutes.

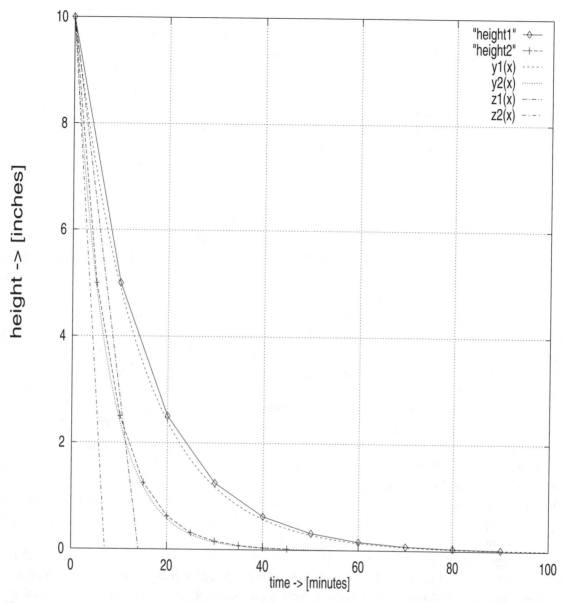

Figure 3–1   A Thought Experiment: The Leaking Bucket of which the Water Level Follows the Same Rules as the Recovery Process

Because these curves have no particular features by which you can easily determine which line belongs to which bucket, you may wonder how to distinguish one smooth curve from another. A straight line that over a very small distance coincides with a curved line is called the "tangential line" of the curve. To distinguish the lines representing the leaking buckets, we draw tangential lines at the beginning of the curves and see where these tangential lines intersect the bottom line, or the time-line. This is the moment in time in which the bucket would be empty if it would keep on leaking at the same rate as it does in the beginning. This corresponds to the moment in time when the bucket is empty if it keeps on leaking at the same fast rate as it does in the beginning. (We know that the leaking slows down towards the end, but if it did continue at the same rate, this moment is when it would be empty.) This moment in time is called the *time constant*.

These smooth, dotted lines have been drawn for both curves. Notice that in Figure 3–1, there are two straight lines going down from the 10-inch height mark on the upper left corner. They are both dash-dot lines, but the right one is dash-dotted tighter than the left one.

These are tangential lines. At the 10-inch mark each of these lines coincides with their curves and go down together at the same rate. The curves, however, veer away from the straight lines, while the straight lines just keep going straight. Notice that the straight line on the right side hits the time-line at the bottom, at approximately 14 minutes, and that the left side straight line hits the timeline near 7 minutes. This is an important point. The slow leaker (the first bucket) has something associate with it that is the time at which the touching line hits the timeline (here 14 minutes) while the twice as fast leaker has a touching line that hits the timeline at 7 minutes: twice as short as 14 minutes!

Thus, you can distinguish these curves from one another by the point where the line that touches them in the beginning hits the timeline. That point is called the *leakage rate time constant*. The first bucket has a leakage rate time constant of 14 minutes, while the second bucket has a leakage rate time constant of 7 minutes. This is important because this is the way in which you can distinguish the different curves you will plot from the exercises in this book.

Another aspect of time curves is shown in Figure 3–2. In this figure, the curve is drawn as a smooth line, starting at time zero, at a value of 100 percent. The tangential line is also drawn in the beginning, and it is noted on the timeline where that tangential line hits it, which is at 1. This point is the time constant for the curve. This kind of curve is so plentiful in nature that scientists have given this time constant its own symbol, represented by τ, the Greek letter for "t" (described as *tau* and pronounced as "tow," which rhymes with "how"). You will notice that the value of the curve at the moment when the tangential line hits the timeline, that is at time τ, is about 37 percent. It is important to note that the curve falls to 37 percent of its starting value after exactly one time constant τ. It is also important to note that the curve falls to 50 percent of its original value when the time that has elapsed is 0.7 times the time constant τ.

One more note: This curve never reaches zero. It approaches zero slowly, but the bucket never is completely empty. Of course, practical people will say that the bucket will be empty at some point. While this is true, the bucket becomes empty because of natural evaporation, which has nothing to do with leakage. However, these practical people are correct. Thus it is important to define the process as having ended (that is, the bucket has been emptied) when the curve has fallen to 1 percent of its starting value. A quick look at the graph reveals that this happens at a moment in time that is 4.5 times the time constant τ.

This is important to the stroke recovery process because *if you can find the curve that represents your recovery, you can predict when you will be fully recovered*. What you must find is the time constant of the recovery process, multiply it by 4.5, and hatsekidee! (pardon my Dutch)—this is the time that you will be back to normal.

COMPLICATIONS

This all sounds wonderful, but certain complications may change this theory and its implementation in an exercise regimen. However, these complications don't change the basic tenet of the method. The basic tenet is twofold:

1. The recovery curves are suitably described by exponential decay functions, and

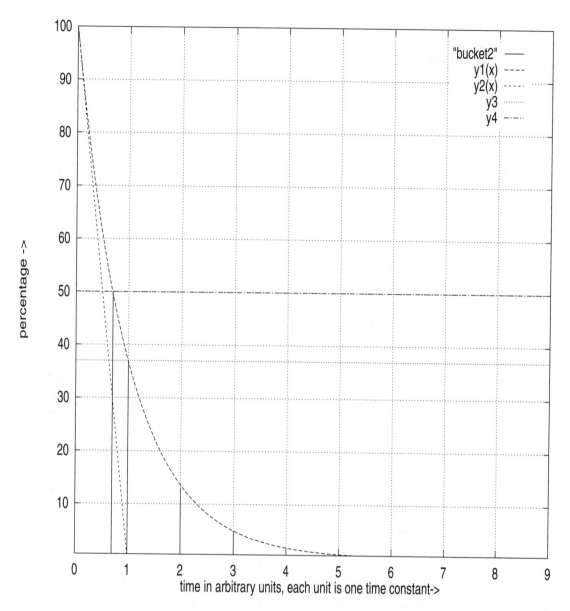

Figure 3–2   Time in Arbitrary Units. Each Unit Is One Time Constant.

2. By measuring how you are doing, you can determine the exponential decay curve for each of your exercises; get to know your improvement rate and your weak points; design an exercise that is structured along the same lines as the many exercises in this book; and improve yourself in weak areas.

Just as in the example of the leaking buckets, complications may arise. In the leaking bucket example, a possible complication may be that the bucket leaks so slowly that it takes several days before it is empty. It may also be impossible to keep all factors consistent all the time—the temperature and humidity, for example, vary from day to day, while the person who measures the height may not do so in exactly the same way each day. This will affect the smoothness of the curve, and may add to it a few bumps that can be easily recognized as caused by daily variations. Likewise, you may not be able to perform your exercises in the same way every day. It could be that your affected hand starts to hurt and you cannot concentrate on the exercise, or you may change an exercise and, as a result, your performance changes. Such changes will show up as deviations from the curve. However, I believe that if the sources of the deviations are removed, the performance will return to the normal recovery process.

WHAT IS NORMAL?

Of course, reality is a bit more complex than this explanation makes it sound. One factor that makes the stroke recovery process different from the leaking bucket example is that the performance you are measuring to determine your recovery is the "correct" performance. It is clear, of course, that if you are measuring how long it takes you to put 10 pencils in a coffee mug (which you will do in Exercise 10), the time it takes never reaches zero. This differs from the measurement of the water level in the bucket, which does reach zero. Instead, when you are recovering, the time it takes to do certain exercises approaches the time it takes for a person with *normal* control over his or her hand to do the same exercises. This is the recovery process: you slowly approach the performance of a normal person. Although you can never do an exercise in zero seconds, the difference between the time it takes you to do an exercise and the time it takes a normal person to do an exercise can reach zero.

Another Example: Where Normal Is Just About Zero

In this book, there are several exercises where you don't measure *how long* it takes you to perform a task, but measure instead *how well* you perform a task. For example, in Exercise 7, you throw a ball in the air with your unaffected hand and catch it with your affected hand. The exercise counts how many times out of 100 throws you miss the catch. (If this sounds difficult, remember that other exercises gradually lead up to it.) A normal person catches all 100 throws, and his or her number of missed catches is therefore zero. Your number of missed catches may be 90 on the first day, but it will gradually reach zero. At that time, you will have reached complete normalcy in this exercise.

QUICK TRICKS AND DIRTY RULES

Some facts about exponential decay curves are also valid for recovery curves. From now on we will refer to the time constant of a recovery curve as the *recovery rate time constant*.

In Figure 3–3 the performance of a normal person is compared with the performance of a stroke patient. The comparison consists of the measurement of how long it takes to perform a certain task. A stroke patient may need a very long time to perform a task, while a normal person performs the task quickly. We call the total difference 100 percent, that is the starting value. After successive repetitions the stroke patients get better and better, approaching the performance of a normal person. Now the difference between the stroke patient and the normal person has shrunk to 0 percent.

Consider this example: Assume you do a particular exercise—say, for example, you are making a fist 10 times in succession. The very first day you do this exercise, it takes you 2 minutes. You keep doing the exercise every day, measuring how long it takes you to make a fist 10 times, and you find that it takes 7 weeks to get this exercise down to 50 percent of its starting time value. So after 7 weeks, you find that the amount of time it takes to make a fist 10 times in a row is now reduced to 1 minute (or reduced to 50 percent of 2 minutes, which is 1 minute). This means that the 0.7 time constant is equal to 7 weeks, or that the time constant is 10 weeks. You can thus expect that if you exercise and take your measurements every day, after 10 weeks, you will do the exercise in 37 percent of 2 minutes, or around 45 seconds.

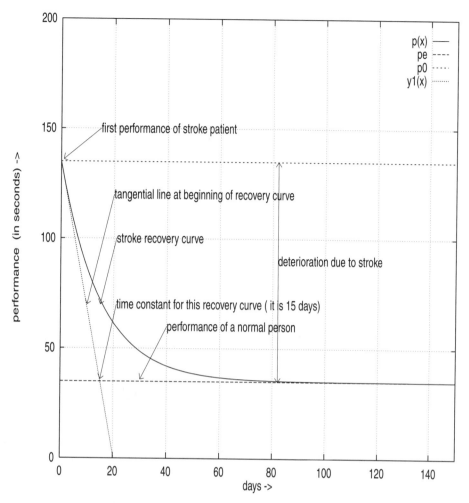

Figure 3–3 Time in Units of Time Constants[1]

DIFFERENT EXERCISES, DIFFERENT TIME CONSTANTS

Our research has shown that recovery occurs at different rates for different exercises. The most striking example is that the recovery rate for a simple exercise, such as catching a ball, is much shorter than that for a five-finger typing exercise. However, both exercises follow an exponential decay curve, only with different time constants for each exercise.

[1]A tangential line is a straight line that over a short distance coincides with a curved line. It does not cross it, but merely coincides with it.

4

The Indispensable Exercise Bike

Exercises on an exercise bike are a must. Researchers have hinted at this, but have not yet definitively documented it,[1] and there remains a certain degree of skepticism about it. However, I discovered by accident what happens if you quit using the exercise bike in terms of your stroke recovery. While I was recovering from my stroke, I did the same exercises every day, improving gradually over three months. Meanwhile, I also exercised on an exercise bike in order to improve my endurance. At a certain point, I thought that my endurance had reached a sufficient level, and decided to switch my 10-minute daily biking exercise with a one-hour walking exercise.

For the first two or three months of this switch, not much happened, although my arm and hand started to become increasingly painful. Then one day I typed my exercise performance numbers in my computer and made a printout of my performance plots. I noticed that instead of showing consistent improvement, I had deteriorated in all exercises—a little in some, quite a bit in others, and dramatically in a few. I had not changed my medication, diet, or the stopwatch I was using. I had not changed the color of paper on which I was writing, or the computer or software I was using. I had not changed the time of day at which I was exercising (always first thing in the morning). I had not changed anything (or so I thought). I was dumbstruck. How could all my exercise times have increased while I had been so diligent? Had I had another small stroke that had gone unnoticed?

I went to my doctor and neurologist to be tested for an unnoticed stroke, but the doctors found nothing. At this point, I panicked. I decided that instead of doing my exercises once a day, I would do them three times a day. With a nervous eye on the graphs, I noticed that indeed, doing exercises three times a day reversed the deterioration, and that I was improving again. I continued with this regimen and saw steady improvement. A few months later, it finally dawned on me that perhaps the problem lay in my having changed from a 10-minute ride on the exercise bike to a one-hour walk in the evening. I looked back at my exercise records and to my astonishment, the day I switched to walking coincided with the day I had started to deteriorate in my other exercises. Realizing the connection, I immediately began exercising on the bike again, and after one week had reduced my times for several exercises by as much as 30 percent. On top of that, the pain in my arm and hand lessened considerably.

Unfortunately, these events don't come with a convenient label that describes their cause and effect. However, using my experience and some educated guesswork, you can deduce that during a one-hour walk, the affected arm dangles passively from the shoulder, while during a 10-minute bike exercise, it is actively engaged in flexing muscles, keeping them supple, and preventing them from stiffening. It is this prevention from stiffening that is crucial to the recovery process. I found that the best bike exercises are those in which little effort is spent; that is, the exercises in which you move a lot but expend little or no force. These exercises keep the arm mobile, are not very tiring, and do not cause exhaustion. This leaves you with energy left over for your other exercises.

I found that walking is not only a bad substitute as an endurance exercise, it also causes the dangling arm to bump against the body at every step, sending a torrent of confusing sensory impulses to the dead part of the brain. Meanwhile, the other parts of the brain, which are busy regulating other body functions, also receive these signals. These other brain parts must figure out what these signals mean, and they become severely overloaded. For me, this resulted in many episodes of painful arm twitches, which felt like I was holding on to a rapidly switching high-voltage cable. I was thus unable to perform my other exercises at full performance level. These episodes of painful arm twitches subsided once I went back to biking exercises.

The moral of this story, therefore, is: **EXERCISE ON A BIKE!**

[1]See for example, Freund, H.J. (1996). Remapping the brain. *Science*, **272**, 1754.

5

Exercise 0: The Bike

Purpose: To enhance endurance and to prevent the stiffening of muscles.

Description: You ride on an exercise bike with hand and foot pedals.

When can you start to do this exercise? In consultation with your physician and therapist, you may be able to start when you are discharged from the hospital.

What do you need for this exercise? An exercise bike that has moving pedals and moving hand grips, preferably the type in which the handgrip and foot-pedal motions are coordinated. The bike must also have an electronic timer and a distance meter. If it has an adjustable resistance implement, make sure that it is set to zero resistance. (I found a bike of this type at a local discount store for 129 dollars. Similar bikes are available for use at local gyms.)

THE EXERCISE: THE FIRST TWO MONTHS

1. Note the date and the day number in the appropriate columns in Table 5–1.
2. For this exercise, you will ride on the bike for a limited amount of time. The time consists of a fixed amount and a variable amount; the fixed amount is 1 minute, the variable amount is 10 seconds times the number of the day. For instance, if this is the first day that you do this exercise, the number of the day is 1. So the first day, the number of seconds that you ride is:

   60 seconds (the fixed amount of time) +10 seconds (the variable amount of time) = 70 seconds (the total amount of time you ride on the bike).

   The second day you ride for 60 seconds + 2 x 10 seconds = 80 seconds; the third day you ride for 60 seconds + 3 x 10 seconds = 90 seconds; and so on. In the course of about two months, your riding time increases to roughly 10 minutes per day.
3. Sit on the bike and make sure that you are comfortable.
4. Start the timer and start riding the bike.
5. When you have been riding for the amount of time appropriate for the given day, look at the distance meter for the ride, memorize the distance, and slowly come to a halt.
6. Get off the bike and record the distance in Table 5–1.

Table 5–1   Table for Distance Bike Exercises

Date	Day #	Time	Distance
/ /			
/ /			
/ /			
/ /			
/ /			
/ /			
/ /			
/ /			
/ /			
/ /			
/ /			
/ /			
/ /			
/ /			
/ /			
/ /			
/ /			
/ /			
/ /			
/ /			
/ /			
/ /			
/ /			
/ /			
/ /			
/ /			
/ /			
/ /			
/ /			
/ /			
/ /			

THE EXERCISE: AFTER THE FIRST TWO MONTHS

After two months, you will be biking 10 minutes every day. You will bike this amount of time for the rest of your recovery period. You are now ready to develop and measure your endurance. To do so, ride the bike for 5 minutes and measure your distance at that time. Then ride the bike for another 5 minutes and record the total distance. If the distance you traveled after 10 minutes is exactly twice the distance you traveled after 5 minutes, it means that you did not slow down during the second 5 minutes. If this is the case, you are in excellent shape. If the distance you traveled after 10 minutes is less than two times the distance you traveled after 5 minutes, you did slow down in the second time interval, which means that your endurance needs improvement.

Follow this step-by-step method to track your endurance.

1. Sit on the bike and start the timer. Ride for 5 minutes. Note the distance you have traveled, and memorize it.
2. Ride for the remainder of the full 10 minutes.
3. Note the distance after 10 minutes and record both this distance and the 5-minute distance you had memorized in Table 5–2 in the column for today under "Distance after 5 Minutes" and "Distance after 10 Minutes."
4. Use your calculator to divide the distance after 10 minutes by the distance after 5 minutes. You should get a number that is in the neighborhood of 2, although it may be a little more or a little less. This number is called the *ratio*. (The word ratio is commonly used to define the result of dividing two numbers.) Record the ratio in the last column in the table.
5. Plot the ratio in the graph on Figure 5–1. Use a small "plus" sign (+) to mark the spot.
6. Plot both the distances in the graph. Use a small circle (o) for the 5-minute distance and a small cross (x) for the 10-minute distance.

If after doing this exercise for two months you find that your 10-minute distance is exactly twice your 5-minute distance, you can quit taking the two time interval distances and just ride the entire 10 minutes, only tracking the final distance. However, it is important that you continue to do this bike exercise for several years, or until you have completely recovered.

Table 5–2   Table for Endurance Bike Exercises

Date	Day Number	Distance after 5 Minutes	Distance after 10 Minutes	Ratio of Two Distances
/ /				
/ /				
/ /				
/ /				
/ /				
/ /				
/ /				
/ /				
/ /				

Table 5–2   Table for Endurance Bike Exercises (*Continued*)

Date	Day Number	Distance after 5 Minutes	Distance after 10 Minutes	Ratio of Two Distances
/ /				
/ /				
/ /				
/ /				
/ /				
/ /				
/ /				
/ /				
/ /				
/ /				
/ /				
/ /				
/ /				
/ /				
/ /				
/ /				
/ /				
/ /				
/ /				

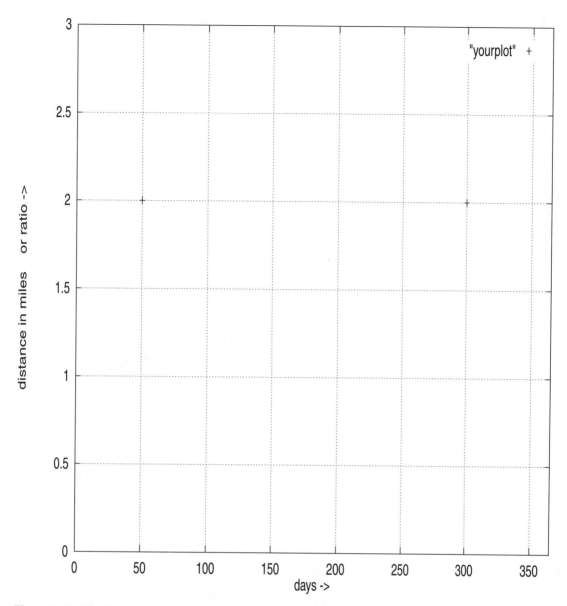

Figure 5–1   Bike Exercise Performance Plot

6

What You Need for the Exercises in This Book

The exercises in this book require very little investment, and most can be done with items readily available in your household. You will need:

1. A spiral-bound notebook to write down your exercise measurements. (Although this book includes a number of tables for this purpose, it is not practical to provide all the space needed for tables in this book.) Many supermarkets and drugstores carry these notebooks. Buy one with at least a hundred pages, as you will need many. It is important that you buy a notebook that lies flat without you having to hold it open.
2. A clear plastic ruler to measure lengths and to draw lines.
3. Ten pencils, or a combination of pencils and pens. Don't use round pencils as they roll away too easily. Ballpoint pens with caps are fine, as are pens with side clips of some sort. Thick pencils and felt-tip pens are easiest to handle.
4. Two large coffee mugs to put pencils in.
5. A cardboard cylinder like those found inside a roll of toilet paper or paper towel.
6. A stopwatch that can be started and stopped, and that retains the time at which it was stopped. It must also be able to restart for the continuation of measurements. You can buy such stopwatches at sporting goods stores.
7. A broom with a stick.
8. A dustpan with a broom.
9. A tennis ball or similar ball, such as a baseball.
10. A typewriter or a computer keyboard. This does not have to be functioning or connected to a computer. You can probably get one for free at a local computer repair shop. Often, repair people wind up with a computer that is beyond repair, and they don't know what to do with the keyboard. They will probably gladly give such keyboards away for free. You can also buy a new keyboard if you wish. I have seen keyboards in the range of 10 to 20 dollars. Choose one that you don't have to push hard on to press the keys. (You don't want to get carpal tunnel syndrome, after all!)

11. A mirror (for face exercises).
12. A telephone handset with the keys in the handset (for thumb exercises). This phone does not have to be connected.
13. A pocket calculator may come in handy for calculating the daily averages of exercises, but is not necessary.
14. A computer with a text processing program for typing exercises in which you count the number of mistyped characters. Does not have to be new.

7

A Complete Exercise Session

This chapter describes a complete exercise session as it worked best for me.

I found that the best exercise with which to start the day was the bike exercise. This exercise warms the muscles and removes the "glue" that forms between the muscle fibers during the night and the previous day. It also stimulates the fingers, arm, thumb, thenar eminens (the bulbous part of the hand where it attaches to the thumb), and legs (one of which was recently paralyzed). In addition, it improves blood circulation. This is important because the circulation in the paralyzed arm is usually poor. (Circulation is caused by motion, which is lacking in the paralyzed arm.) Before you begin your bike exercise, hold your hands next to each other and note any color or temperature difference. A hand with poor circulation appears bluish and puffy and is colder than an unaffected hand, which has a normal pink appearance. Check your hands again after the bike exercise; the affected hand may still be blue and puffy, but it will have warmed up.

When you are ready to start the exercise series, the following sequence is recommended. (These exercises will all be covered in this book.)

1. **Cardboard Cylinder.** This is a medium-fine motor control exercise.
2. **Ten Pencils, Mug-to-Mug.** This is a grasping exercise. It is rather easy, so you may be able to abandon it in a month or so, and concentrate on a more difficult exercise.
3. **Ten Pencils, Mug-to-Table-to-Mug.** This is a grasping exercise, similar to the one mentioned above. This is probably the toughest exercise in the book because it requires extremely gentle treatment; otherwise, the pencils will fall from your fingers. Remember: Only strong people can force themselves to be gentle.
4. **Turn a Pencil Clockwise.** This is an exercise for finer motor control, but it is much easier than Ten Pencils, Mug-to-Table-to-Mug, in which one often drops the pencil.
5. **Turn a Pencil Counterclockwise.** This is an exercise for finer motor control. In this exercise, it is not that important that you hold onto the pencil because you put it down immediately.
6. **Ten Pencils, Eraser-End First.** This exercise is similar to the previous one, only in this exercise you put pencils in a mug with their eraser-end first. This presents two added difficulties: You must cock your wrist while holding the pencil, and your hand partially obscures

the mug. This requires you to think about the spatial relationship between the pencil and the mug.

7. **QW.** This is a typing exercise in which you press letters in pairs. It is the perfect start for individual finger exercises.
8. **QWT.** This exercise is the natural follow-up to the QW exercise.
9. **THREE.** This exercise is the natural follow-up to the QWT exercise.
10. **FOUR.** This exercise is the natural follow-up to the THREE exercise.
11. **FIVE.** This is the last exercise in this series.
12. **WAFERS10/MONOPOLY10.** In this exercise, you type a word with one hand.
13. **The Quick Fox.** In this exercise, you type an entire sentence with both hands to promote coordination.
14. **Racecar.** In this exercise, you type an entire sentence with one hand.
15. **Streetdress.** In this exercise, you also type an entire sentence with one hand.
16. **Philosopher.** In this exercise, you type a poem as fast as you can with both hands.
17. **Medieval Monk.** In this exercise, you type a six-line poem, in which no typos are allowed.
18. **Thumb to Joints.** This is an exercise for the thumb.
19. **Twenty-Nine Facial Exercises.** These are exercises for the face.
20. **One Ball, 1 Foot.** A preparatory ball catching exercise, which you may learn fast.
21. **Catch the Bouncer.** This is the easiest of the ball-catching exercises.
22. **Ball from Left to Right.** In this exercise, you throw and catch a ball with two hands.
23. **Ball Back in Hand.** In this exercise, you throw and catch a ball with the affected hand only.

It initially took me between one and two hours to complete an entire exercise session. This time gradually decreased to an hour due to the fact that every exercise went faster, or became unnecessary and was therefore skipped.

8

How to Make Something Crooked Look Straight

The subject at hand, how to make something crooked look straight, is usually the territory of lawyers, politicians, and orthodontists. But occasionally, scientists must perform acts of "optical illusion" as well. The act of illusion alluded to in this chapter is the changing of axes on a graph so that they appear different yet are still the same. As an example, see Figure 8–1, which is the now-familiar plot of the water level in the leaking bucket.

Note that the line in this plot is curved. Notice also that after one time constant, the value has dropped to 37 percent, and that after two time constants the value has dropped to 13 percent. This is 37 percent of 37 percent. After three time constants, the value has dropped to 5 percent, or 37 percent of 37 percent of 37 percent. For each lapse of time equal to one time constant, the value drops to 37 percent of the amount at the beginning of that time lapse.

Now imagine that the piece of paper on which this plot has been printed is flexible, like a thin sheet of rubber. Imagine that the rubber is not equally thick everywhere, but that it is thickest near the top and thinnest near the bottom. Now imagine that you grab the top edge in one hand and the bottom edge in the other hand, and that you stretch the sheet. Due to the difference in thickness, it will not stretch uniformly; the bottom part will stretch more than the top part does, because the top part is more rigid.

The plot that is printed on the sheet will be deformed, and will look something like the plot in Figure 8–2.

Notice that the curved, printed line now looks like a straight line. The numbers on the axes for each of the points are still there. By stretching the sheet, the original curved line, the exponential decay curve has been transformed into a straight line and you have created a *logarithmic plot*. In this logarithmic plot, the bottom has been stretched more than the top. Not all curves will be straightened out by this transformation, but the exponential decay curve will be. (Although a few other factors have also been changed, they are not important in regards to this book.)

Also note that in the original plot, which is called a *linear plot*, the distance between two points on the vertical axes that are spaced one unit from each other (for example, the distance between 1 and 2) is the same between any two similarly spaced units (for example, it is the same as the distance

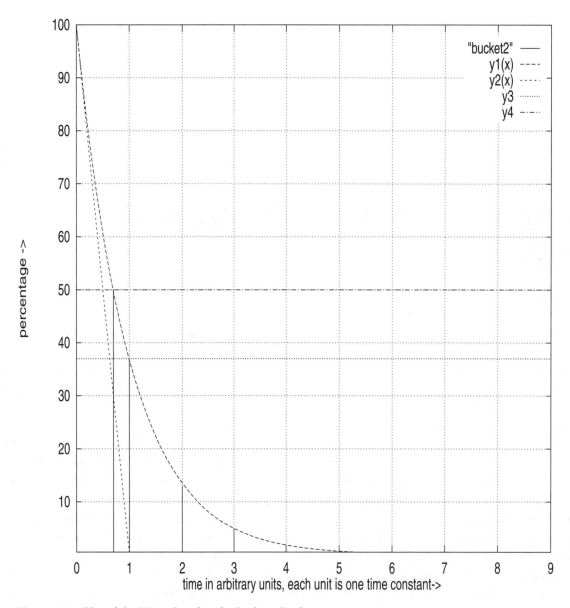

Figure 8–1   Plot of the Water Level in the Leaking Bucket

between 5 and 6); that is, one unit. On the logarithmic plot, this is different. Here, two points on the vertical axis that have a certain ratio to one another (such as a factor of two) have the same distance. To observe this, take a ruler and measure the distance from 1 to 10. You will note that these numbers have a ratio of 10. Now, measure the distance from 10 to 100. You will note that these numbers all have the same factor of 10, and the same distance in this plot. Now, measure the distance from 1 to 100 (that is, a factor of 100). Notice that this distance is twice the distance between 1 and 10 (that is, two factors of 10.) Two factors of 10 is one factor of 100.

Also note that the positions on the vertical line are different. The number zero is absent, while the numbers 20 through 90 have not been printed. Only the numbers 1, 10, and 100 are printed. The first horizontal line above the line that has the number 1 printed in front is the line for the number 2; the line above that is the line for the number 3; above that is the line for the number 4; and so on. There is a line for all numbers between 1 and 10.

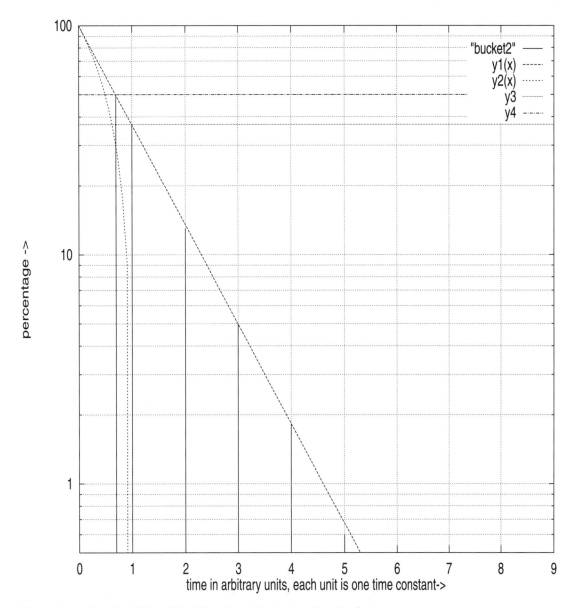

Figure 8–2　Stretched Plot of the Water Level in the Leaking Bucket

Now measure the distance between lines 2 and 4 and between lines 4 and 8, notice that they have the same ratio (2) and the same distance on the plot.

The first horizontal line above the line that has the number 10 in front of it, is the line for 20, above that is the line for 30, above that is the line for 40, and so on. Again, measure the distance from lines 1 to 2 and from lines 10 to 20. Notice that it is the same distance. Also measure the distance from lines 5 to 10 and from lines 10 to 20. They also have the same distance, which is a factor of 2.

If you are interested in reading more about these plots, you can find more information in most high-school-level math books, many of which are available in local libraries.

9

How to Record and Plot Your Data

Recording your data on plots is extremely simple, but there is one pitfall: It is not easy to use the day's date when you are making plots. It is much simpler to number the days and use the day number. However, this also creates an ambiguity, because every exercise has its own starting day. I made a mistake by choosing the starting date for every exercise as day 1 for that exercise. In this way, I wound up with eighteen different day 1s, for eighteen different exercises. This made it difficult to compare exercise performances on given days, since they all had different starting dates. To avoid this problem, **choose as day 1 the FIRST day of the FIRST exercise**. For example, if the first day of the first exercise is 10/10/00, then October 10, 2000 is day 1 for all exercises. If the first day of the second exercise is two weeks later, on 10/24/00, then that exercise starts on day 14; thus, the second day of the second exercise, 10/25/00, is day 15.

USING A STOPWATCH AND A GRAPH

Electronic stopwatches indicate the time in minutes, seconds, and hundredths of seconds. Ignore those hundredths of seconds completely—don't even attempt to round off to the nearest whole number. This is not important enough to waste time on. Record all times in seconds. If an exercise lasts several minutes, convert the entire time into seconds. Remember that 1 minute contains 60 seconds, so that for example, an exercise that lasts 5 minutes 28 seconds lasts:

5 x 60 seconds + 28 seconds = 300 seconds + 28 seconds = 328 seconds.

For each exercise there is an empty plot in which you can make your own graph. If you have never made a plot before, refer to Figure 9–1. This plot is similar to the previous plots. On the bottom there is a horizontal line with numbers printed under it. On the left there is a vertical line with numbers printed on the left of it. The horizontal and vertical lines, called the horizontal axis and the vertical axis, are where you plot the number of the day and your performance. Along the horizontal axis you measure the number of days; therefore, this line is also called the "days" axis. Along the vertical axis you measure your performance; therefore, this line is also called the "performance" (or "seconds") axis. The numbers under the horizontal axis run from left to right, starting with "0" on the left and ending with 350 on the right. (Actually, the horizontal axis extends to 365, the number of days in a full year.) Every 50 days a faint vertical line, a "grid" line, is drawn. These vertical grid lines make it easier to determine positions on the plot.

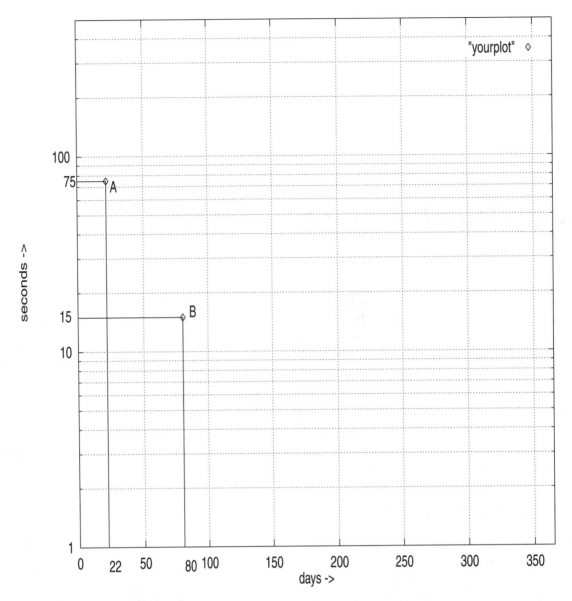

Figure 9–1 Sample Plot Graph

Now look at the vertical axis (the performance axis). To the left, the numbers 1, 10, and 100 have been printed. Look now at the horizontal line that has been drawn next to the number 10. The line underneath it has no number next to it, but it is the line for number 9. Underneath this line is another line, also without a number next to it. That is the line for number 8. Underneath the line for number 8 is the line for number 7, and so on. In the same way, the line above number 10 is the line for number 20, above it is the line for number 30, and so on.

Imagine that on day 22, you do an exercise. The result of your performance (the time it takes you to complete the exercise) is 1 minute 15 seconds, or 75 seconds. In order to plot your performance on the graph, you must make a mark for day 22 at 75 seconds. Because day 22 is not indicated on your sample graph, you must guess where it would be. In this case, it is almost halfway between days 0 and 50. In Figure 9–1, a vertical line and the number 22 have been printed where day 22 would be on the horizontal axis if it had a mark of its own. The number 75 and a horizontal line have also been printed next to the vertical axis where 75 seconds would be if it had a mark of its own.

Now imagine that on day 80, you do another exercise, which takes you 15 seconds to complete. In order to plot your performance on the graph, you must make a mark for day 80 at 15 seconds. Again, because day 80 is not indicated on your sample graph, you must guess where it would be. In this case, it is a little over halfway between days 50 and 100. In Figure 9–1, a vertical line and the number 80 have been printed where day 80 would be on the horizontal axis if it had a mark of its own. The number 15 and a horizontal line have also been printed next to the vertical axis where 15 seconds would be if it had a mark of its own.

For more information on determining averages and time constants, please see Appendix IV.

10

Exercise 1: The Statue of Liberty

Purpose: This exercise helps you begin to move your fingers.
Description: By relaxing the muscles of which you have control and concentrating on those over which you do *not* have control, the fingers are encouraged to move.
When can you start to do this exercise? When you can move your arm and wrist.
What do you need for this exercise? A quiet room and a good chair in which you can sit comfortably.

THE EXERCISE

In this exercise you will sit in an easy chair in a room without distractions (no radio, TV, pets, family members, friends, neighbors, or lovers—all by yourself). This exercise will take up to 30 minutes, so make sure that you can complete it at your leisure and that you schedule no activities before the exercise has ended. For the purposes of this exercise, it is assumed that your left side is paralyzed. If your right side is paralyzed, exchange the left for right in the following instructions.

In order to begin the exercise, you must first get rid of the leftover strain in your muscles. You can do this by contracting and releasing the muscles over which you have control. For instance, if your right side is not affected, you can relax it by contracting every muscle on that side, and then releasing the contraction. By putting a small amount of strain on a muscle and then letting it go, you force the muscle to relax. If you do not first contract the muscle, strain will be left over in it from previous activities. This is important because in this exercise, your brain is trying to control muscles over which it does not yet have control. The last thing it needs is to receive messages from muscles that have nothing to do with the current task at hand.

Sit down, take a deep breath, and begin your relaxation process. Begin with your eyes, open and close them lightly three times, at a medium strength three times, and then open and close them lightly again three times. Your eyes should now be relaxed. Now, relax your forehead. Raise your eyebrows three times just a little bit, then three times as high as you can, and then again three times a little bit.

Now gently frown three times. Then, frown a medium stern frown three times, and finish with three gentle frowns. To make sure that at the end there is no trace of the frown left over, raise your eyebrows gently three times. This process is now repeated in the same way for the other muscles of your face (if you have control over them). Relax all muscles in the same way: three gentle contractions, three medium-strength contractions, and three gentle contractions again. Complete this for the following facial motions:

1. Smile.
2. "Pout" your lips.
3. Open your mouth.
4. Pull up your nose and upper lip.
5. Pull down your lower lip.
6. Pull back your ears (This is important for people who wear glasses because a sweaty face causes glasses to slide down. These people often use their ears to pull their glasses back into a normal position. If you don't wear glasses, feel free to skip this part.)

Now move on to your right arm. Normally, to move a body part, you need two muscles: one to move it and the other to move it back. Do the following movements three times lightly, three times with medium force, and three times lightly again:

1. Move your shoulder forward.
2. Move your shoulder backward.
3. Move your shoulder upward.
4. Lift your arm up and down at your sides.
5. Lift your arm up and down in front of you.
6. Bend your elbow.
7. Straighten your elbow.
8. Bend your wrist inward.
9. Bend your wrist outward.
10. Bend your fingers.
11. Touch your thumb to the tip of your little finger.

Remember that this is not an athletic exercise but a relaxation exercise, so move as gently as you can, and make sure that the muscle you are working on is relaxed before you start on the next one.

You are now ready to work on your right leg. Do these motions again in the same pattern: three times lightly, three times with medium force, and then three times lightly again:

1. Lift your knee.
2. Push your heel back against a chair.
3. With your heel on the floor, lift you toes.
4. With your toes on the floor, lift your heel.
5. Turn your foot inward.
6. Turn your foot outward.

Do the same exercises using your left leg.

You are now ready to work on your left arm (the affected arm). Using the same pattern (three times lightly, three times with medium force, and then three times lightly again):

1. Flex your elbow (if you can).

2. Bend your wrist inward.
3. Bend your wrist outward.

All the muscles over which you have control should now be relaxed. If you still feel tense, apply the same motions to the applicable muscles. You will now have spent approximately 20 to 30 minutes getting relaxed. It is now time to begin the next part of the exercise.

In this part of the exercise, you will actually move your fingers. First, lightly touch the muscles that control the fingers of your affected hand with the fingers of your unaffected hand. These muscles are located on the inside of your forearm. Next, put both hands in your lap and relax completely again. Slowly make a fist with your unaffected hand and, at the same time, make a fist with your affected hand and SQUEEZE, SQUEEZE, SQUEEZE—as hard as you can. (Don't forget to breathe!) At the same time, watch very carefully what happens to the fingers on your affected hand. Did they move? If they did, you are on your way to recovery. If they did not move, don't be discouraged; try again tomorrow. Keep on trying until you see your fingers move ever so slightly. Once you see your fingers move, continue with this exercise every day for a week.

Examples and Experiences

This exercise was inspired by a discussion I had with my sister-in-law, Yvonne Smits-Ruijsink, who is a physical therapist living in The Hague, in the Netherlands. She explained to me the details of this exercise, which is based on a technique called *autogenic training*. It took me about 35 minutes to complete the first time, and the result was that I saw just a tiny bit of movement in my fingers.

In order to complete the exercise, I imagined my body as a large building in the shape of a body—like the Statue of Liberty in the New York harbor—only seated, like I was at that moment. Inside the building were narrow and wide hallways, stairways, and passages through which I could walk. Lofts, elevator shafts, and openings in the floors allowed me to pass from one floor to another. In all of these hallways were ducts, water- or oil-filled hoses, hydraulic presses, fans, motors, steel tension cables, pulleys, bellows, conveyor belts, and so on. There were also loudspeakers, video monitors, surveillance cameras, and equipment for measuring such things as the temperature and humidity. Deep inside the building were conduits for electrical cables, phone cables, fiber optic links, and intercoms.

I walked around the building; in some areas it was very busy, and in others it was eerily quiet. In the quiet areas I felt the palpable atmosphere of suspended action. I checked all the meters, and put my foot on the hoses to gauge their pressure. I felt for tension in the wires, knocked on the ducts to see if they were clogged, and smelled the air. I noted that although everything was in perfect working order, some pieces of equipment in certain wings of the building did not work, although nothing was physically wrong with the equipment. The problem, I noticed, was that no signals were reaching the equipment because a partial breakdown had occurred in the top-floor control room of the building. In the Statue of Liberty, this room is inside the space where the spikes emanate from the head. I called this room the brainroom.

Inside the brainroom, technicians were frantically trying to rewire the messed-up signals. Part of their problem was that the measuring equipment—surveillance cameras, microphones, thermometers, pressure sensors, all the equipment they needed to check new wire connections—did not respond. This was because this equipment was also connected to the non-functional part of the brainroom. They had to try many times to see if a new wiring scheme would work. Some of the technicians sent messengers out of the control room into the building to see if a new wiring connection had had any effect. Others hung out of the top-floor windows trying to look inside the windows on a floor below. Occasionally, I heard a euphoric roar in the control room when they found a way to repair a piece of equipment or signal.

My task was to pinpoint a particular nonworking apparatus, which the control crew would then try to restart. I would put my hand on a motor, feel its slight vibrations, and send a telepathic brainwave up to the crew in the brainroom. They would then pick up this brainwave, and quickly change some wires to see if doing so had any effect. If it did, I would let them know, again by telepathic brainwave, and would go on to a new piece of equipment. You can imagine the relief of the crew when one day, a creaking, heaving sound was heard, and the Statue of Liberty moved her previously debilitated hand and fingers.

As it was my job to make sure that everything in the building was working properly, I had to open all doors and check every room. The building was used for various purposes. In one room I saw a group of people in wheelchairs swapping stories about how miserable they were, and how much they wanted to be back to normal. This was apparently a stroke recovery support group. In an adjoining room I saw a group of disability insurance lawyers busy trying to find out how they could squirm from under their obligation to pay benefits to the patients next door. In a third room, I saw officials of the Social Security Administration busy denying benefits (in this case, to a legal resident alien, even though he had paid social security premiums much longer than the required 40 quarters, not to mention that he had paid his taxes like any American). In another room I saw an exhausted woman trying to comfort her paralyzed husband, who thought that he might never be normal again.

Finally, in yet another room I saw a woman sitting in an easy chair, all by herself, with no radio or TV on. She had a book with a spiral back on the floor next to her. Although I had no idea what she was doing, I felt a vague sense of familiarity with her. I imagined that she was imagining that her body was a large building in which there were many rooms that she was walking through. I imagined that she had just walked into a room in which she saw a man sitting all by himself, with no radio or TV on, no pets, family, or friends, all by himself. . . .

11

Exercise 2: Rub a Surface

Purpose: To stimulate sensation in the hand.
Description: Rub the hand over a variety of surfaces with different roughness and textures.

THE EXERCISE

At the end of this chapter you will find a list of many materials and geometrical shapes, each with its own surface structure. In this exercise, you will identify places in your home where you these materials or shapes are located, and rub your hand over them for 3 to 4 seconds. By doing so, you will stimulate the sensory system in your hand so that you will begin to feel more. As you rub each surface, check them off in this book (if you can carry it with you). Try to feel the texture, shape, and temperature of the surfaces. Also try to feel the difference between cool, warm, and lukewarm surfaces. Try do determine where the actual feeling is occurring—on your fingertips, on the shafts of your finger, in the palm of your hand, or on the skin of the thenar eminens (the bulbous part of your hand where it attaches to the thumb). Carefully pay attention to what you feel and where you feel it. Do this exercise every day until you find that there are no clear distinctions between the rubs of today and the rubs of yesterday. Then you can safely quit this exercise.

The list of surfaces is as follows. At the bottom of the list there are a few open spaces where you can fill in your own favorite surfaces.

1. Wool (such as that found on a jacket or sweater)
2. Cotton (such as that found on a blouse or shirt)
3. Flannel (such as that found on a shirt or pajamas)
4. Formica (such as that found on a kitchen counter)
5. Metal (such as that found on a refrigerator door)
6. Linoleum (such as that found on floor tiles)
7. Wallpaper
8. Painted wood (such as that found on a door)
9. Plastic
10. Unpainted wood (such as that found on kitchen cabinet doors)

11. Glass (such as that found on a drinking glass or bottle)
12. Window glass
13. Gabardine (such as that found on a suit or jacket)
14. A floor rug
15. Leather (such as that found on a shoe or chair)
16. Cotton from a bathroom towel
17. The fur of your dog or cat (if you have one)
18. Your own hair (or your bald head, as the case may be)
19. Wicker from a basket or furniture
20. Something round (such as a dough pin or a table leg)
21. Something with a sharp edge (such as a kitchen counter or a door jamb)
22. A newspaper
23. A magazine
24. Human skin (your own, your spouse's, or that of a friend)
25.
26.
27.

12

Exercise 3: A Broomstick Clock

Purpose: This exercise trains the hand to rotate an object while holding on to it in different orientations.

Description: To train the hand to hold an object and rotate it in space.

When can you start to do this exercise? When you can close your fist. (Discuss this exercise with your physician or your therapist before you start, to make sure that you can safely do it.)

What do you need to do this exercise? You will need a broom with a stick.

THE EXERCISE

When you close your fist for the first time, you will notice that all your fingers will bend simultaneously. (You have already done this in Exercise 1.) In this exercise, you will close your hand around a stick, such as broomstick. For the purposes of this exercise, it is assumed that your left side is paralyzed. If your right side is paralyzed, exchange the left for right in the following instructions. To complete the exercise, perform the following steps:

1. Take the broomstick in your hand and hold it vertically, with the broom portion on the bottom.
2. Move the broom so that your arm is fully forward, then fully sideways. Move it this way 10 times. (Be careful not to hit anybody with the broom, while you do this.)
3. Imagine that the top of the broomstick is the small hand of a clock. When you hold it vertically, the top of the broomstick points upwards, or in the direction of 12 o'clock. Hold it in this position with your arm **fully forward**.
4. Now rotate the broomstick (not your arm!) so that it points in the direction of 1 o'clock. Return to the 12 o'clock position.
5. Now rotate the broomstick to the 1 o'clock position and continue to the 2 o'clock position. Now return to the 1 o'clock and 12 o'clock position.
6. This time, try to move forward again, all the way to 3 o'clock. Each time the broomstick is in a full-hour position, pause for a few seconds before moving forward.
7. When you reach the 3 o'clock position, return to the 12 o'clock position, only this time move further back to the 11 o'clock and 10 o'clock positions.

8. Try to move on to the 9 o'clock position. When you have reached the 9 o'clock position, go forward to the 3 o'clock position again. Each time the broomstick is in a full-hour position, pause for a few seconds before moving forward.
9. Now perform this exercise with your arm **fully sideways** instead of fully forward. In this case, don't go all the way to the 9 o'clock or 3 o'clock position because you may hurt your shoulder. Stop when it becomes uncomfortable.

Repeat this exercise three times a day for two to three weeks. You may then have enough control over your hand to quit this exercise.

13

Exercise 4: Push Yourself Back from a Wall

Purpose: This exercise increases upper arm strength.
Description: Push yourself back from a wall.
When can you start to do this exercise? When you can safely stand on your feet and bend over without falling. (Discuss this exercise with your physician or your therapist to make sure that they agree that you can do this exercise safely.)

THE EXERCISE

1. Stand facing a wall at a distance of about 2 feet.
2. Place the palms of your hands against the wall roughly at eye level.
3. Now carefully lean over and touch the back of your **affected** hand with your forehead.
4. Push yourself back until you are straight on your feet again, then lean over and touch the back of your **unaffected** hand with your forehead again.
5. Lean forward again, touching each hand with your forehead 10 times.

When you are done with this exercise you should feel that your triceps (the muscles on the backside of your upper arms) are working, and may even hurt a little. By working these muscles, you are using your affected hand together with your unaffected hand to increases upper arm strength. You should perform this exercise every day for about two to three weeks.

14

Exercise 5: One Ball, 1 Foot

Purpose: This exercise trains the affected hand in holding onto a ball that falls into it.

Description: In this exercise, you drop a ball into your affected hand and try to grasp it. The ball falls approximately 1 foot in distance before it is caught.

When can you start to do this exercise? When you can move your hand in such a way that the palm is facing up, and when you can grasp a ball dropped into your palm so that it does not roll out of your hand.

What do you need for this exercise? You need a ball that fits in your hand. A tennis ball or a baseball are perfect examples. (A golf ball is probably too small unless you have very small hands). Test the size by holding the ball in your unaffected hand. There should be a space of about 1/2 to 2 inches between the tip of your thumb to the tip of your ring finger. The ball does not have to be covered with felt or leather. You may choose to use a sand-filled toy-balloon that you can knead, which you may choose to do as an exercise. These balls are often sold at drugstores and novelty stores. They are not perfectly round, so they are a bit more difficult to catch.

THE EXERCISE

1. Write the date and the day number in the "Date" and "Day #" columns of Table 14–1.
2. Take the ball in your unaffected hand and stretch out your unaffected arm.
3. Stretch your affected arm out with the palm of your hand turned upward, so that your affected hand is about 1 foot below the ball.
4. Drop the ball into your affected hand and try to catch it.
5. Do this 100 times and count how many times you are unable to catch the ball. (This sounds very simple, but this exercise has a hidden pitfall: the counting is confusing. You have to keep track of two varying numbers: the number of times you have dropped the ball into your hand and the number of times you were unable to hold onto it. This is confusing enough for people who have not had a stroke and who have no problems with their brain, but stroke survivors have a problem with their hands as well as with their brain, and therefore may have trouble counting. Don't feel ashamed if you lose count or don't catch the ball.

Here is one way to keep your counting straight: First, say aloud the number of times you dropped the ball in your hand, then say "and," and then say the number of times you were unable to hold onto the ball. You thus say aloud two numbers and the word "and" every time you drop the ball into your affected hand. Saying the count aloud makes it easier to keep track, because you still "hear" in your head which numbers you said if there is an interruption. This is especially important if you drop a ball and it rolls away and you have to go look for it. By the time you get back, you may have forgotten how many times you caught or missed the ball.

6. When you have dropped the ball 100 times into your hand, record the number of times you were unable to hold onto it in the column labeled "Number Missed" in Table 14–1. If you have set a record today, congratulations! Record your score in the column labeled "Records."

7. Plot the number of times you missed catching the ball in the graph in Figure 14–1.

8. Plot the number of times you missed catching the ball in the "Overall Perspective Plot" in Chapter 36.

Table 14–1   One Ball, 1 Foot Exercise Table

Date	Day #	Number Missed	Records
/ /			
/ /			
/ /			
/ /			
/ /			
/ /			
/ /			
/ /			
/ /			
/ /			
/ /			
/ /			
/ /			
/ /			
/ /			
/ /			
/ /			
/ /			
/ /			
/ /			
/ /			
/ /			

Table 14–1   One Ball, 1 Foot Exercise Table (*Continued*)

Date	Day #	Number Missed	Records
/ /			
/ /			
/ /			
/ /			
/ /			
/ /			
/ /			
/ /			
/ /			

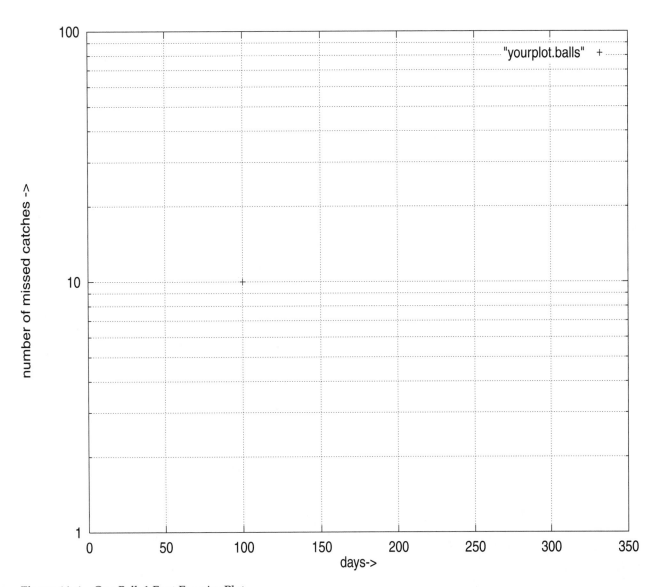

Figure 14–1   One Ball, 1 Foot Exercise Plot

Discussion

In the beginning you may find that you must react very quick, and you may be a little wary that the quick jerky motion you must make in order to catch the ball may be bad for you. Discuss this with your physician or therapist. They will be best able to help you determine how well this exercise suits you needs.

Examples and Experiences

I did this exercise mostly standing. I found that I mastered it rather quickly—in a week or so—although I did experience that the sudden dropping of the ball was sometimes—especially in the beginning— a bit too jerky for me.

15

Exercise 6: Catch a Bouncer

Purpose: This exercise trains the affected hand in speed and precision and also improves hand-eye coordination.

Description: In this exercise, you drop a ball from your affected hand to the floor and catch it on the rebound.

When can you start to do this exercise? You can start to do this exercise when you can move your hand so that the palm faces up, and when you can grasp a ball so that it does not roll out of your hand. You must also be able to stand and bend your knees without falling.

What do you need for this exercise? You need a ball that fits in your hand and that bounces well, such as a tennis ball. (A golf ball is probably too small unless you have very small hands.) Test the size by holding the ball in your unaffected hand. There should be a space of about 1/2 to 2 inches between the tip of your thumb to the tip of your ring finger. For this exercise, a sand-filled toy-balloon does not work well because it doesn't bounce. To make sure your ball bounces well, drop it from a height of 3 feet onto a hard floor. If it bounces up to around 1 foot, then it has the right bounce. In most cases, a ball like those sold in drugstores (usually with a plastic baseball bat) will also work.

THE EXERCISE

1. Write the date and the day number in the columns "Date" and "Day #" in Table 15–1.
2. Stand with your feet firmly on the floor, with about 1 1/2 feet between them.
3. Bend your knees somewhat, so that your body is a little lower than usual.
4. Put the ball in your affected hand and tilt your hand so that the ball rolls out of it and falls onto the floor.
5. Catch the ball on its rebound while it is at its highest point.
6. If you caught the ball, congratulations—you are on your way to recovery. If you missed it, try again.
7. Repeat this exercise 100 times.

8. Count how many times you have bounced the ball and how many times you have missed catching it on the rebound. (See Exercise 5 for helpful hints on counting, as this can be confusing.)

9. Record the number of times you missed catching the ball in the "Number Missed" column in Table 15–1. If you have set a record today, congratulations! Record your score in the column labeled "Records."

10. Plot the number of times you missed catching the ball in Figure 15–1.

11. Plot the number of times you missed catching the ball in the "Overall Perspective Plot" in Chapter 36.

Table 15–1   Catch a Bouncer Exercise Table

Date	Day #	Number Missed	Records
/ /			
/ /			
/ /			
/ /			
/ /			
/ /			
/ /			
/ /			
/ /			
/ /			
/ /			
/ /			
/ /			
/ /			
/ /			
/ /			
/ /			
/ /			
/ /			
/ /			
/ /			
/ /			
/ /			
/ /			
/ /			
/ /			
/ /			
/ /			

Table 15–1   Catch a Bouncer Exercise Table (*Continued*)

Date	Day #	Number Missed	Records
/ /			
/ /			
/ /			
/ /			
/ /			

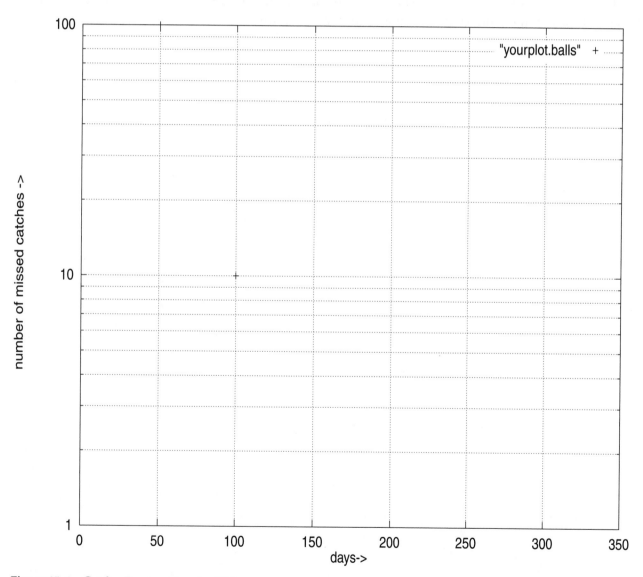

Figure 15–1   Catch a Bouncer Exercise Plot

Discussion

I advise that you bend your knees quite a bit in this exercise so that your back remains more or less straight while you are catching the ball. It is also a good idea to support your body by placing your unaffected hand on your knee on your unaffected side. Before you start with the exercise, swing your hips to make sure that you have good balance. If you have trouble standing and keeping your balance, you may want to discuss this exercise with your doctor or a therapist. You may choose to skip this exercise altogether—there are plenty of other exercises in this book that you can do without compromising your balance. Be careful when you bend and spread your legs or when you make quick movements in this exercise; you do not want to fall and hurt yourself.

Examples and Experiences

This exercise is challenging, yet it is one that you can master in a few days. Scooping up the ball in the air can be exhilarating, especially since you have spent much of your time recovering from your stroke in hospitals, in rehab centers, in wheelchairs, and maybe in intensive care—and now you are catching balls! I missed catching the ball 12 times out of one hundred on the first day and reduced this to 2 times on the tenth day. After that, I discontinued this exercise.

16

Exercise 7: Ball from Left to Right

Purpose: This exercise trains the affected hand in speed and precision and improves hand-eye coordination. It also stimulates blood circulation in the affected arm and hand.

Description: In this exercise, you throw a ball into the air with your unaffected hand, catch it with your affected hand, and then throw it back to the unaffected hand.

When can you start to do this exercise? You can start to do this exercise when you can move your hand so that the palm faces up, and when you can grasp a ball so that it does not roll out of your hand. You must also be able to stand and bend your knees without falling. (These are the same requirements as for the previous exercise, but they are less stringent for this exercise because you don't have to bend over.)

What do you need for this exercise? For this exercise you need a ball that fits in your hand, such as a tennis ball or baseball. (A golf ball is probably too small unless you have very small hands.) Test the size by holding the ball in your unaffected hand. There should be a space of about 1/2 to 2 inches between the tip of your thumb to the tip of your ring finger. For this exercise, a sand-filled toy-balloon works well since no bouncing is required. In fact, if you have used a perfectly round ball for a few weeks, change over to the sand-filled toy-balloon, as it is not perfectly round and is therefore slightly more difficult to catch.

THE EXERCISE

1. Write the date and the day number in the columns "Date" and "Day #" in Table 16–1.
2. Stand with your feet firmly on the floor, with about 1 1/2 feet between them. Your foot on the affected side should be slightly in front of your unaffected foot.
3. Take the ball in your unaffected hand and throw it up in the air and catch it with your affected hand.
4. If you have caught it, congratulations—you are on your way to recovery. Throw it back to your unaffected hand and repeat the throw. If you missed it, pick it up and start over.
5. Repeat this exercise 100 times.
6. Count how many times you have thrown the ball and how many times you have missed it. (See Exercise 5 for helpful hints on counting, as this can be confusing.)

7. After 100 throws, record the number of missed balls in the "Number Missed" column in Table 16–1. If you have set a record today, congratulations! Record your score in the column labeled "Records."
8. Plot the number of times you missed catching the ball in Figure 16–1.
9. Plot the number of times you missed catching the ball in the "Overall Perspective Plot" in Chapter 36.

Table 16–1   Ball from Left to Right Exercise Table

Date	Day #	Number Missed	Records
/ /			
/ /			
/ /			
/ /			
/ /			
/ /			
/ /			
/ /			
/ /			
/ /			
/ /			
/ /			
/ /			
/ /			
/ /			
/ /			
/ /			
/ /			
/ /			
/ /			
/ /			
/ /			
/ /			
/ /			
/ /			
/ /			
/ /			
/ /			
/ /			
/ /			

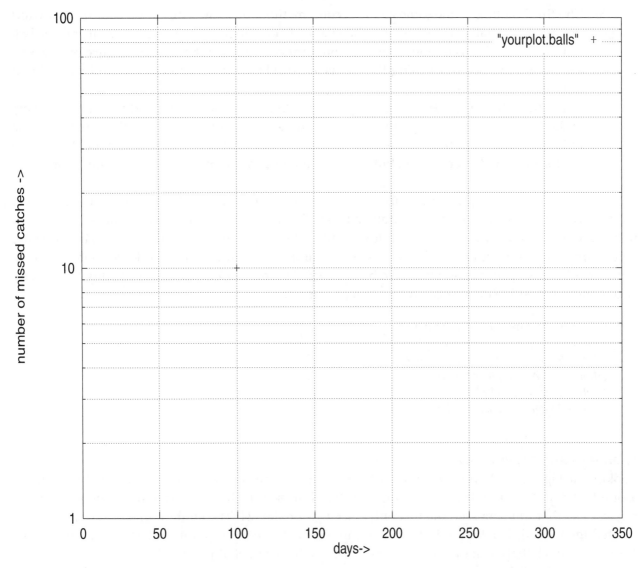

Figure 16–1   Ball from Left to Right Exercise Plot

Discussion

As in the previous exercise, if you have trouble standing and keeping your balance, you may want to discuss whether you should do this exercise with your doctor or therapist. However, the demands on your balance are fairly light, so you may want to give it a try.

This is a complex exercise, and you will find that there are several ways to catch the ball:

1. The first method is to form a cup with your hand and quickly move the cup into the trajectory of the ball so that the ball falls into it. You may find that the ball frequently bounces out of the cup.
2. The second method is to form a cup with your hand and let the ball bounce off the inside of your fingers and into the bottom of the cup. In this method you touch the ball with your hand twice, and are more likely to catch it.

3. The third method is the same as the second method, but now you move your hand toward you while the ball bounces against the inside of your fingers. By doing this, you *grab* the ball out of the air. This is a more active catching process and you have more chance of success.
4. The fourth method of catching the ball is to quickly bend your fingers around the ball and hold it.
5. The fifth method is an extension of the fourth. In this method, you bend your middle, ring, and little fingers, and squeeze the ball between these three fingers and the thenar eminen (the bulbous part of your hand at the base of your thumb). Often, the index finger and the thumb are too slow to do very much, but with this method you improve your catching ability.

Such catching techniques may sound extremely trivial to someone who has not had a stroke, yet for a stroke patient who is partially paralyzed, catching a ball is a difficult task. This exercise is an important one because you not only improve your ability to move your hand, you also improve the blood circulation in your arm and develop better hand-eye coordination. Hand-eye coordination is important because your vision may have been affected by the stroke; hence your ability to estimate speed and the position of objects may have been impaired.

On a Border Guard Evader with a Stroke
In El Paso there lived an old smuggler
whose life story was that of a struggler
but he said "A ball from left to right?
I will practice day and night
Because I might get a job as a juggler."

Examples and Experiences

Looking at Figure 16–2 you can see that I missed 20 catches on the first day and that it took me around 10 days to reduce the number of times that I missed the ball to half of that number, or to 10 misses. The first time I missed the ball only once was on day 24. The straight line is a computer-calculated (generated) line that indicates the minimum distance to all points; it has a time constant of 159 days. Notice that the more I did this exercise, the better I got at it.

I found that this was a pleasant, somewhat hypnotic exercise, and it often put me in a relaxed mood. This exercise was also terrific for the affected arm, which got a real workout.

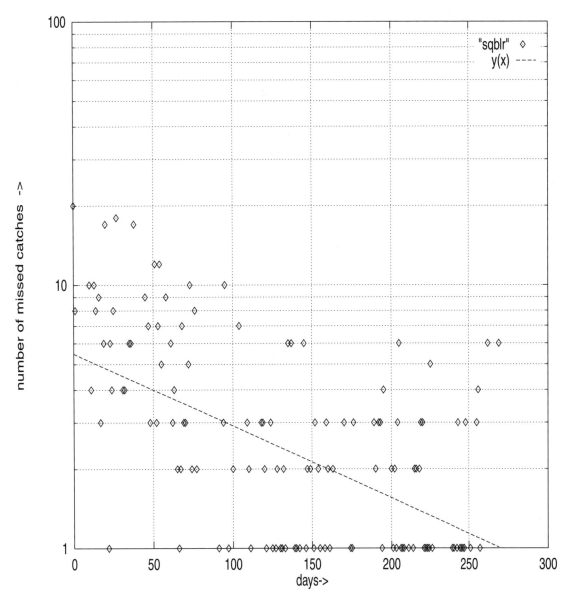

Figure 16–2   Plot of Author's Performance in Ball from Left to Right Exercise

17

Exercise 8: Ball Back in Hand

Purpose: This exercise trains the affected hand in speed and precision and improves hand-eye coordination. It also stimulates blood circulation in the affected arm and hand.

Description: In this exercise, you repeatedly throw a ball in the air with the affected hand, catching it in the same hand.

When can you start to do this exercise? You can start to do this exercise when you can move your hand so that the palm faces up, and when you can grasp a ball so that it does not roll out of your hand. You must also be able to stand and bend your knees without falling. (These are the same requirements as for the previous exercise, so you can do this exercise if you could do the previous one. However, it is wise to start this exercise a few days or a week after you start the previous exercise in order to get used to the motions.)

What do you need for this exercise? You need the same ball that you used for the previous exercise.

THE EXERCISE

1. Write the date and the day number in the columns "Date" and "Day #" in Table 17–1.
2. Stand with your feet firmly on the floor, with about 1 1/2 feet between them. Your foot on the affected side should be slightly in front of your unaffected foot.
3. Take the ball in your affected hand, throw it up in the air, and catch it with your affected hand.
4. If you have caught it, congratulations—you are on your way to recovery. Throw it back up and catch it again. If you missed it, pick it up and start over.
5. Repeat this exercise 100 times.
6. Count how many times you have thrown the ball and how many times you have missed it. (See Exercise 5 for helpful hints on counting, as this can be confusing.)
7. After 100 throws, record the number of missed balls in the "Number Missed" column in Table 17–1. If you have set a record today, congratulations! Record your score in the column labeled "Records."
8. Plot the number of times you missed catching the ball in Figure 17–1.

9. Plot the number of times you missed catching the ball in the "Overall Perspective Plot" in Chapter 36.

Table 17–1 Ball Back in Hand Exercise Table

Date	Day #	Number Missed	Records
/ /			
/ /			
/ /			
/ /			
/ /			
/ /			
/ /			
/ /			
/ /			
/ /			
/ /			
/ /			
/ /			
/ /			
/ /			
/ /			
/ /			
/ /			
/ /			
/ /			
/ /			
/ /			
/ /			
/ /			
/ /			
/ /			
/ /			
/ /			
/ /			

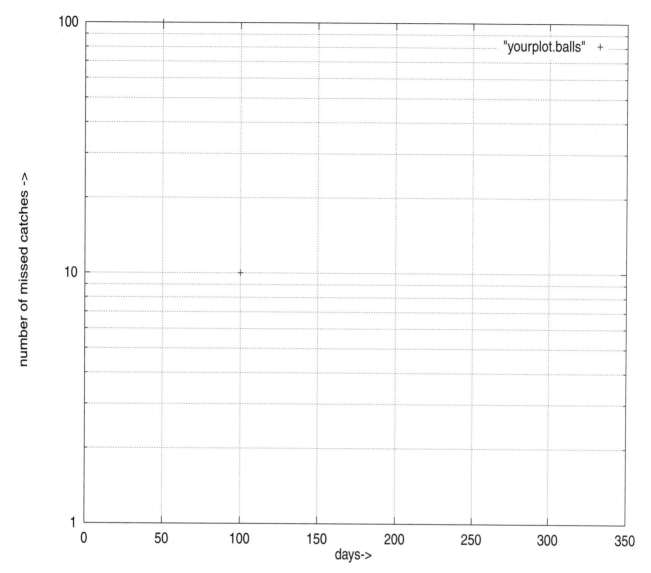

Figure 17–1   Ball Back in Hand Exercise Plot

Discussion

As in the previous exercise, if you have trouble standing and keeping your balance, you may want to discuss whether you should do this exercise with your doctor or therapist. However, the demands on your balance are fairly light, so you may want to give it a try. Please see Exercise 7 for hints on various methods of catching the ball.

This exercise is more difficult and much faster than the previous one was. It is such a fast exercise that you may get tired rather quickly. It is a good idea to not throw the ball too high, in order to avoid making wild rescue swings if the ball goes a little off course. Such sudden movements are not good for you. Throwing the ball to around shoulder height is best.

Examples and Experiences

Looking at Figure 17–2 you can see that it took me around 210 days to reduce the number of times that I missed catching the ball from 29 (on the first day) to 3.5 (the average between 3 on some days,

4 on others, on day 210). My score kept on going down, although with great daily fluctuations. The first day I had a perfect score was on day 19 (not shown here because a zero cannot be shown in a logarithmic plot). Notice that the recovery rate time constant was measured to be 146 days by determining how long it took to reduce the average score by a factor of two and then multiply by 1.4 (See Appendix IV). Notice also that it took me until day 104 to get my score consistently down in the neighborhood of 2 to 3 missed catches per 100. Notice also that the more I did this exercise, the better I got at it.

Because there is a considerable amount of luck involved in catching a ball after throwing it in the air 100 times, you can never really tell if you have mastered this exercise. Only through a statistical analysis can you tell where you are in the recovery process. I kept on doing this exercise longer than was necessary because I felt that it was also good for my blood circulation. Every morning when

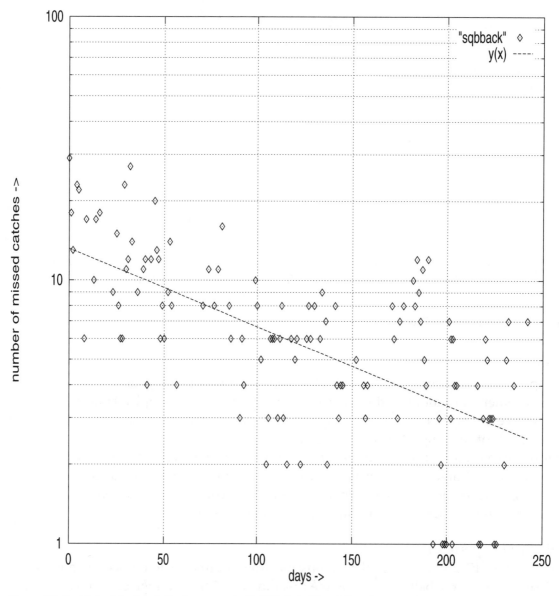

Figure 17–2   Plot of Author's Performance in Ball Back in Hand Exercise

I woke up, I noticed that my affected hand was bluer than my unaffected hand was due to poor circulation. I therefore felt that it was important to keep my arm moving as much as I could.

Variation on a Theme: Exercise 8–2: Ball Back in Hand on One Foot

After a while, you may get really good at catching the ball, missing maybe 5 or 8 out of 100 throws. At this time, you may want to add a degree of difficulty that will require more physical activity. This will improve your general physical condition as well.

In this variation, you stand on one foot (the foot of your affected side) and do the very same exercise as described above. (You should discuss this exercise with your doctor or therapist; be extremely careful when you start any exercise or variation.) Before beginning this exercise, shift your weight to your foot on your affected side and touch the ground with your toes on your unaffected side. If you feel you are properly balanced, lift your unaffected foot and stand on your affected foot only. Perform the exercise and record your score in the same way as you did before, adding a vertical line in the plot to indicate the day you changed the exercise. You will notice that your score (the number of missed balls) will go up drastically because you now have to pay attention to four things:

1. Maintaining your balance. (This is not easy!)
2. Catching the ball.
3. The number of throws you have made.
4. The number of balls you have missed.

I recently heard that circuses have had to cut costs, and that they have replaced the strong man with a man with strong character. When you feel you have mastered this exercise, you may want to consider applying to the circus for a job as a somewhat paralyzed juggler!

18

Exercise 9: Cardboard Cylinder

Purpose: This exercise trains the hand in grasping a medium-size object.

Description: In this exercise you place a cardboard cylinder in a flower vase or large bowl.

When can you start to do this exercise? You can start to do this exercise when you can grasp a relatively thick cylinder (roughly 1 1/2 inches thick).

What do you need for this exercise? For this exercise you need a relatively thick cardboard cylinder (such as those found inside a roll of toilet paper or paper towels). Paper towel cylinders are preferable because they are longer. You will also need a flowerpot (vase or bowl) in which the cardboard cylinder can be placed without it falling out. You will also need a stopwatch.

THE EXERCISE

1. With your unaffected hand, start the stopwatch.
2. With your affected hand, put the cylinder in the pot, and let go of it. Take the cylinder back out and place it on the table.
3. Repeat this exercise 30 times, counting like this: 1 in, 1 out, 2 in, 2 out, 3 in, 3 out, 4 in, 4 out, and so on.
4. When you reach 30 out, stop the stopwatch with your unaffected hand.
5. Record the time in Table 18–1.
6. Plot your time in Figure 18–1.
7. Plot your average time in the "Overall Perspective Plot" in Chapter 36.

Discussion

This exercise prepares you for upcoming exercises in which you train your fine motor control. (The thicker cardboard cylinder used in this exercise is easier to grasp than a pencil or ballpoint pen, which you will use in later exercises.) Make sure that you grasp the cylinder between your index finger and thumb, and not with your full hand. Try to keep the middle, ring, and little fingers away from the cylinder. This way, you manipulate the cylinder only with your thumb and index finger. You will probably get the hang of this exercise in a couple of weeks, after which you may go on to the next exercise.

Table 18–1   Cardboard Cylinder Exercise Table

Date	Day #	Number Missed	Records
/ /			
/ /			
/ /			
/ /			
/ /			
/ /			
/ /			
/ /			
/ /			
/ /			
/ /			
/ /			
/ /			
/ /			
/ /			
/ /			
/ /			
/ /			
/ /			
/ /			
/ /			
/ /			
/ /			
/ /			
/ /			
/ /			
/ /			
/ /			
/ /			
/ /			
/ /			

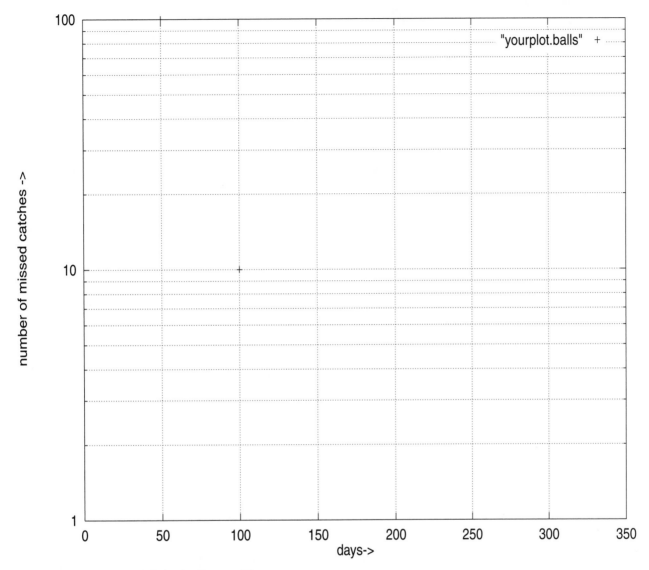

Figure 18–1   Cardboard Cylinder Exercise Plot

19

Exercise 10: Ten Pencils, Mug-to-Mug

Purpose: This exercise trains the affected hand to move medium-sized objects.

Description: In this exercise, you put 10 pencils in a mug, and then put them one by one into another mug.

When can you start to do this exercise? You can start to do this exercise when you can touch the tip of your thumb to the tip of your index finger.

What do you need for this exercise? For this exercise you need two large coffee mugs, 10 pencils or a combination of pencils, ballpoint pens, and felt-tip pens. (Do not use round pencils or pens, as they roll away too easily. Pens with caps or side clips will also work, as will six-sided pencils. Make sure that the tips are dull so that you do not hurt yourself.) You will also need a stopwatch that can be started, stopped, and restarted.

THE EXERCISE

1. Place the two mugs side by side in front of you. (We will call them Mug 1 and Mug 2.)
2. With your unaffected hand, put the 10 pencils in Mug 1. Make sure that they are spread out evenly around the mug, as you would put flowers in a vase.
3. With your unaffected hand, start the stopwatch.
4. With your affected hand, take the first pencil out of Mug 1 and put it in Mug 2. Continue to take individual pencils out of Mug 1 and put them in Mug 2. If the pencils tend to bunch up in Mug 1, separate them with your unaffected hand. (It is difficult to pick up individual pencils if they are bunched up.) If you drop a pencil, just pick it up with your unaffected hand and put it in Mug 2.
5. When you have put all pencils in Mug 2, stop the stopwatch.
6. With your unaffected hand, spread all the pencils out evenly in Mug 2.
7. Restart the stopwatch with your unaffected hand.
8. With your affected hand, remove all pencils from Mug 2 individually, and put them in Mug 1.
9. Stop the stopwatch when you have put all the pencils in Mug 1.
10. Read the stopwatch time and record it under the "Required Time #1" column in Table 19–1.

11. Repeat steps 2 through 9 and record your time under the "Required Time #2" column in Table 19–1.
12. Repeat steps 2 through 9 for a third time and record your time under the "Required Time #3" column in Table 19–1.
13. Calculate the average of the three required times and record it under the "Average" column in Table 19–1. If you have set a record today, congratulations! Record your score in the column labeled "Records."
14. Plot your average time in Figure 19–1. (See Chapter 9, "How to Record and Plot Your Data," for directions on plotting your data in the graph.)
15. Plot your average time in the "Overall Perspective Plot" in Chapter 36.

Table 19–1   Ten Pencils, Mug-to-Mug Exercise Table

Date	Day #	Required Time #1	Required Time #2	Required Time #3	Average	Records
/ /						
/ /						
/ /						
/ /						
/ /						
/ /						
/ /						
/ /						
/ /						
/ /						
/ /						
/ /						
/ /						
/ /						
/ /						
/ /						
/ /						
/ /						
/ /						
/ /						
/ /						
/ /						
/ /						
/ /						
/ /						
/ /						

Table 19–1 Ten Pencils, Mug-to-Mug Exercise Table (*Continued*)

Date	Day #	Required Time #1	Required Time #2	Required Time #3	Average	Records
/ /						
/ /						
/ /						
/ /						
/ /						
/ /						
/ /						
/ /						
/ /						
/ /						
/ /						
/ /						
/ /						
/ /						
/ /						
/ /						
/ /						
/ /						
/ /						
/ /						
/ /						
/ /						
/ /						
/ /						
/ /						
/ /						
/ /						
/ /						
/ /						
/ /						
/ /						
/ /						
/ /						
/ /						

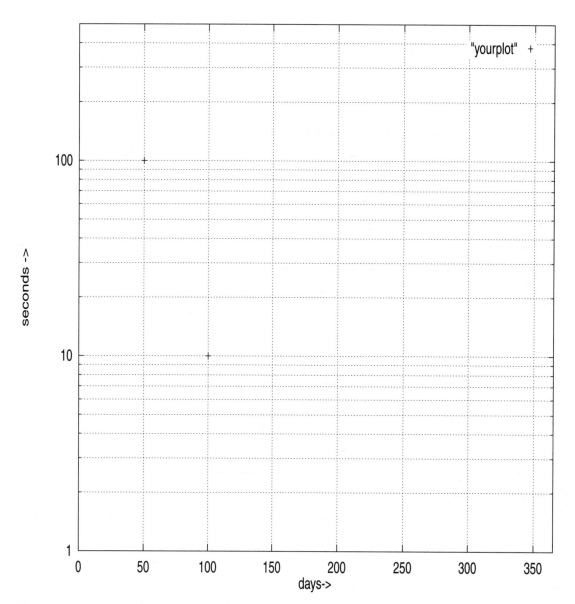

Figure 19–1   Ten Pencils, Mug-to-Mug Exercise Plot

20

Exercise 11: Ten Pencils, Mug-to-Table-to-Mug

Purpose: This exercise trains the affected hand to pick up medium-sized objects.

Description: In this exercise, you put 10 pencils in a mug, remove them individually, place them on the table, and put them back in the mug.

When can you start to do this exercise? You can start to do this exercise when you can pick up a relatively thick cylinder (such as a magic marker or a felt-tip pen) from a table.

What do you need for this exercise? For this exercise you need a coffee mug, 10 pencils or a combination of pencils, ballpoint pens, and felt-tip pens. (Do not use round pencils or pens, as they roll away too easily. Pens with caps or side clips will work, as will six-sided pencils. Make sure that the tips are dull so that you do not hurt yourself. You may be best off using relatively thick pens, as thinner pencils are difficult to grasp.) You will also need a stopwatch that can be started, stopped, and restarted.

THE EXERCISE

1. Place the mug in front of you. With your unaffected hand, put all 10 pencils in the mug. Make sure that they are spread out evenly around the mug, as you would put flowers in a vase.
2. With your unaffected hand, start the stopwatch.
3. Take the first pencil out of the mug with you affected hand, and place it on the table. Continue to take the pencils out one at a time, placing them on the table.
4. When all the pencils have been removed, stop the stopwatch.
5. The pencils are now jumbled on the table. With your unaffected hand, put them all neatly next to one another so that you can pick them up without having to touch other ones.
6. Restart the stopwatch with your unaffected hand.
7. Pick up the first pencil, hold it for a second or two, and move your hand towards the mug. When you reach the mug, point the pencil down into the mug. When it is completely inside the mug, let it go. (This sounds very simple, but it is actually difficult. If you are unable to

pick the pencil up, don't worry about it. Try again with something thicker than a pencil, such as a marker.)

8. Repeat this step for the next pencil, separating it from the other pencils on the table to facilitate grasping it. Continue this process until all the pencils are in the mug.
9. Stop the stopwatch when you have put all the pencils back in the mug.
10. Record the time in the "Required Time #1" column in Table 20–1.
11. Repeat steps 1 through 9 and record your time in the "Required Time #2" column in Table 20–1.
12. Repeat steps 1 through 9 for a third time and record your time in the "Required Time #3" column in Table 20–1.
13. Calculate the average of the three times and record it under the "Average" column in Table 20–1. If you have set a record today, congratulations! Record your score in the column labeled "Records."
14. Plot your average time in Figure 20–1. (See Chapter 9, "How to Record and Plot Your Data," for directions on plotting your data in the graph.)
15. Plot your average time in the "Overall Perspective Plot" in Chapter 36.

Table 20–1   Ten Pencils, Mug-to-Table-to-Mug Exercise Table

Date	Day #	Required Time #1	Required Time #2	Required Time #3	Average	Records
/ /						
/ /						
/ /						
/ /						
/ /						
/ /						
/ /						
/ /						
/ /						
/ /						
/ /						
/ /						
/ /						
/ /						
/ /						
/ /						
/ /						
/ /						
/ /						
/ /						
/ /						

Table 20–1   Ten Pencils, Mug-to-Table-to-Mug Exercise Table

Date	Day #	Required Time #1	Required Time #2	Required Time #3	Average	Records
/ /						
/ /						
/ /						
/ /						
/ /						
/ /						
/ /						
/ /						
/ /						
/ /						

Discussion

Despite the apparent simplicity of this exercise, it is actually quite difficult. When I tried to do it for the very first time, it took me more than 5 minutes to complete. Even many months later, after at least 200 times trying to do it, I was often unable to complete it.

The first way in which your hand learns to grasp an object is the "lateral pinch." In this motion, the thumb touches the side of your index finger to facilitate picking up an object. This is not the same as the "opposing pinch" in which the soft, fleshy part of the tip of the thumb touches the soft, fleshy part of the index finger to grip an object.

The exercise is difficult because the space between the table and the curvature of the skin of the finger and the thumb is small. If you try to pick up the pencil and exert too much force, you squeeze the pencil out of the space between your finger and thumb, and it remains on the table. Another problem is that your thumb tends to bend rather than remain straight; this causes the thumbnail to touch the pencil, which results in your not being able to hold it. Meanwhile, your thumb moves upward, sliding alongside the finger; this rolls the pencil away from you. You can avoid this by exerting only a minimum amount of force. You are also likely to become frustrated when you cannot pick up the pencil; as a result, you may pinch too hard and be less capable of picking it up.

The exercise is also difficult because your other fingers may want to bend when you are trying to pick up the pencil with your thumb and index finger. There are many such "associative movements" in which in moving one muscle, you move another as well. Think of people lifting something heavy; their face contorts with the effort. This is the result of "neural overflow." This occurs when the neural impulses on one nerve required to move a muscle are also felt on another nerve and thus move another muscle. In this exercise, the bending of the index finger causes the middle finger to bend as well. Just when you think that you have the pencil firmly grasped, your middle finger pushes it away. To avoid this, pay extra attention to where your middle finger is. Try to keep its side touching the side of your index finger. That way, it will follow the movement of the index finger, making it less likely to knock the pencil out of your grasp. It also helps to be as gentle as you can when you pick up the pencil, because the less force you exert with your index finger, the less associative movement there will be with your middle finger.

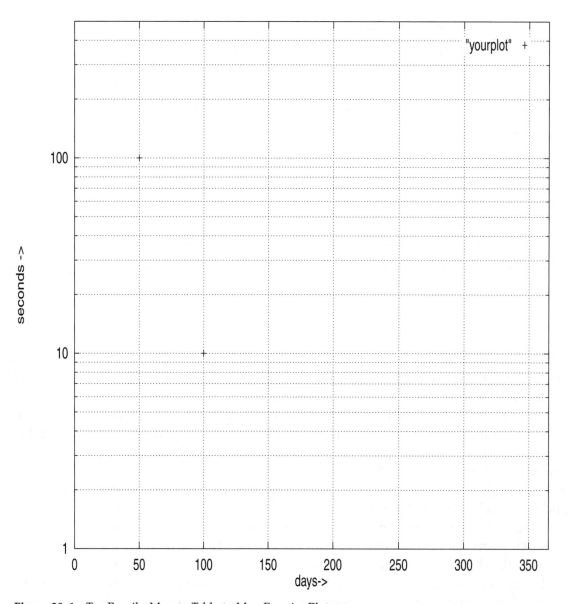

Figure 20–1   Ten Pencils, Mug-to-Table-to-Mug Exercise Plot

Since this is a difficult exercise, you should expect variations in the time it takes you to perform it. On some days I could not do it at all, while on other days I was more successful. If you cannot do this exercise, try exercising with the cardboard cylinder for a few weeks, then try this exercise again. Also note that it is best not to wash your hands before doing this exercise because sweaty hands make picking up the pencil easier.

A stroke patient complained from his bed
"I will certainly wind up dead
'cause these exercises
are full of surprises,
I now have to fill my cup with wood and lead"

Examples and Experiences

As you can see in Figure 20–2, I showed initial improvement when I began doing this exercise, but experienced a dramatic deterioration. After roughly 200 days, I dropped the pencil more and more frequently, and had a hard time finishing the exercise. I found that my middle finger often pushed the pencil out of my grasp (due to bending from neural overflow). I thus had to do the cardboard cylinder exercise for three months before I could go back to this exercise. (I did the cardboard exercise from days 200 to 300. I put the cardboard cylinder in a vase 30 times and divided the required time by 3 to get a measurement similar to the Ten Pencils, Mug-to-Table-to-Mug exercise.) As you see, once I got the hang of the exercise again, I improved. After roughly two years I decided that my performance had probably leveled off to that of a normal person, and I quit doing the exercise. (As you can see in Figure 20–2, after day 600 there are a few days that it took me an unusually long time to complete the exercise. This is because I had taken a sleeping pill the night before.)

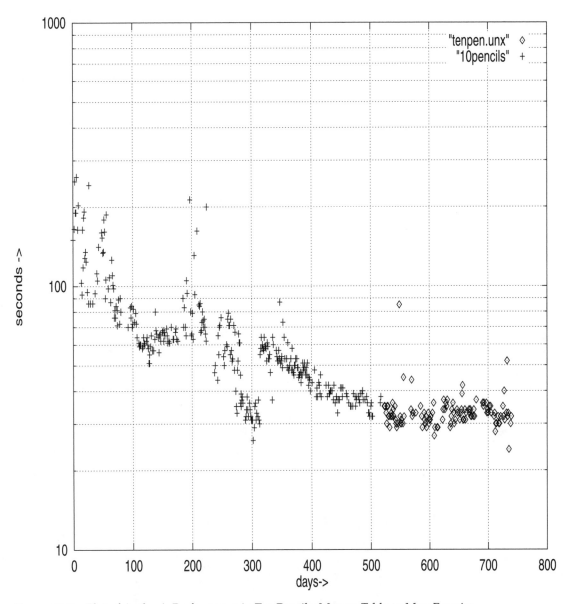

Figure 20–2   Plot of Author's Performance in Ten Pencils, Mug-to-Table-to-Mug Exercise

21

Exercise 12: Turn a Pencil Clockwise

Purpose: This exercise trains the affected hand to grasp an object and rotate it clockwise. (This motion is needed when you turn doorknobs, turn on and off faucets, etc.)

Description: In this exercise, you put a pen or pencil on the table with the tip away from you, pick it up and turn it clockwise, and put it down with the tip towards you.

When can you start to do this exercise? You can start to do this exercise when you can stretch out your affected hand with your palm up and turn it so that your palm is facing down, and when you can pick up a pencil from a table.

What do you need for this exercise? For this exercise you need a relatively thick pencil or felt-tip pen (about as thick as your index finger) with a cap in a different color (for ease of distinguishing the tip from the other end). You will also need a stopwatch that can be started, stopped, and restarted.

THE EXERCISE

1. With your unaffected hand, start the stopwatch.
2. With your unaffected hand, put the pencil with its tip away from you on the table. With your affected hand pick it up and turn it towards you in a clockwise direction, and put it back on the table. (That was a half turn.) Pick the pencil up again with your affected hand, turn it in a clockwise direction, and put it down with the tip away from you. (That makes one whole turn.) Repeat this for 10 whole turns (20 half turns).
3. When you have completed 10 whole turns (20 half turns), stop the stopwatch with your unaffected hand.
4. Read the stopwatch time and record it under the "Required Time #1" column in Table 21–1.
5. Repeat steps 1 through 4 and record your time under the "Required Time #2" column in Table 21–1.
6. Repeat steps 1 through 4 for a third time and record your time under the "Required Time #3" column in Table 21–1.
7. Calculate the average of the three required times and record it under the "Average" column in Table 21–1. If you have set a record today, congratulations! Record your score in the column labeled "Records."

8. Plot your average time in Figure 21–1. (See Chapter 9, "How to Record and Plot Your Data," for directions on plotting your data in the graph.)
9. Plot your average time in the "Overall Perspective Plot" in Chapter 36.

Table 21–1   Turn a Pencil Clockwise Exercise Table

Date	Day #	Required Time #1	Required Time #2	Required Time #3	Average	Records
/ /						
/ /						
/ /						
/ /						
/ /						
/ /						
/ /						
/ /						
/ /						
/ /						
/ /						
/ /						
/ /						
/ /						
/ /						
/ /						
/ /						
/ /						
/ /						
/ /						
/ /						
/ /						
/ /						
/ /						
/ /						
/ /						
/ /						
/ /						
/ /						
/ /						
/ /						
/ /						

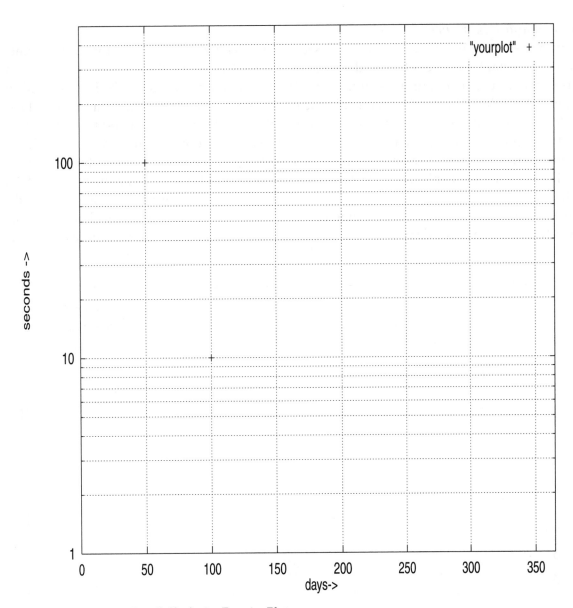

Figure 21–1   Turn a Pencil Clockwise Exercise Plot

Discussion

This exercise is a variation on Exercise 11, with two added difficulties: the clockwise rotation, and the releasing of the pencil from a rotated hand. Opening the hand is always more difficult than is closing it, and now you have to open it in a rotated position, which is even more difficult than it is in a normal position. This exercise is useful because the motion is a part of many aspects of daily living, such as turning a doorknob, turning a faucet on and off, twisting the cap off a bottle, and turning a key in a lock.

> *A carpenter whose main utensils*
> *for turning table legs were steel stencils*
> *said "No big deal,*
> *it's just my spiel,*
> *to recover, I will turn pencils."*

Examples and Experiences

As you can see in Figure 21–2, it took me 42 seconds to complete the exercise for the first time. This is a very important exercise; I had to do this exercise for two years, three times a day. The hardest part is to make sure that your index finger and thumb do not bend too much. They should remain straight and parallel to each other, with only the tips moving. This is very difficult because it requires the extenders and the flexors (the muscles that straighten and bend the fingers) to work at the same time. It may take months before you can do it. I had a similar problem in this exercise as I had in the previous exercise; namely, my middle finger pushed the pencil away from me (due to neural overflow). I don't have any explanation for my deterioration around day 280. Fortunately, the deterioration disappeared soon after it appeared. The straight line is a computer-drawn calculation of the best fitting line through all points; it has a time constant of 700 days. Of course, this line does not accurately reflect the behavior of my recovery, as the real recovery process is much more complex.

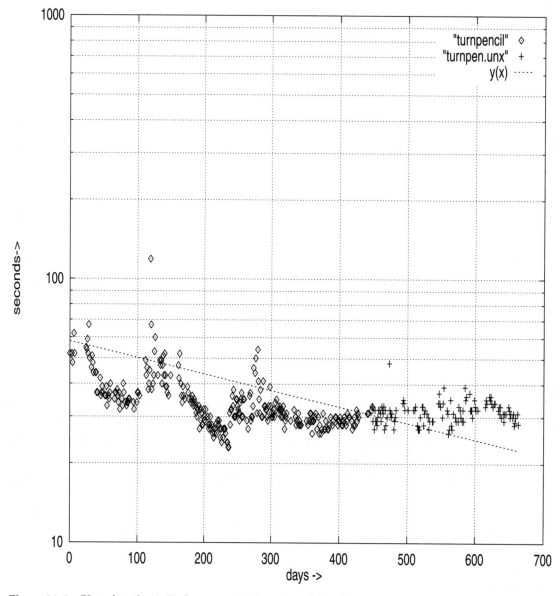

Figure 21–2   Plot of Author's Performance in Turn a Pencil Clockwise Exercise

22

Exercise 13: Turn a Pencil Counterclockwise

Purpose: This exercise trains the affected hand to grasp an object and rotate it counterclockwise. (This motion is needed when you turn doorknobs, turn on and off faucets, etc.)

Description: In this exercise, you put a pen or pencil on the table with the tip away from you, pick it up and turn it counterclockwise, and put it down with the tip towards you. This exercise is like the previous one except that you turn the object in the opposite direction.

When can you start to do this exercise? You can start to do this exercise when you can stretch out your affected hand with your palm up and turn it so that your palm is facing down, and when you can pick up a pencil from a table.

What do you need for this exercise? For this exercise you need a relatively thick pencil or felt-tip pen (about as thick as your index finger) with a cap in a different color (for ease of distinguishing the tip from the other end). You will also need a stopwatch that can be started, stopped, and restarted.

THE EXERCISE

1. With your unaffected hand, start the stopwatch.
2. With your unaffected hand, put the pencil with its tip away from you on the table. With your affected hand pick it up and turn it towards you in a counterclockwise direction, and put it back on the table. (That was a half turn.) Pick the pencil up again with your affected hand, turn it in a counterclockwise direction, and put it down with the tip away from you. (That makes one whole turn.) Repeat this for 10 whole turns (20 half turns).
3. When you have completed 10 whole turns (20 half turns), stop the stopwatch with your unaffected hand.
4. Read the stopwatch time and record it under the "Required Time #1" column in Table 22–1.
5. Repeat steps 1 through 4 and record your time under the "Required Time #2" column in Table 22–1.
6. Repeat steps 1 through 4 for a third time and record your time under the "Required Time #3" column in Table 22–1.

7. Calculate the average of the three required times and record it under the "Average" column in Table 22–1. If you have set a record today, congratulations! Record your score in the column labeled "Records."
8. Plot your average time in Figure 22–1. (See Chapter 9, "How to Record and Plot Your Data," for directions on plotting your data in the graph.)
9. Plot your average time in the "Overall Perspective Plot" in Chapter 36.

Table 22–1   Turn a Pencil Counterclockwise Exercise Table

Date	Day #	Required Time #1	Required Time #2	Required Time #3	Average	Records
/ /						
/ /						
/ /						
/ /						
/ /						
/ /						
/ /						
/ /						
/ /						
/ /						
/ /						
/ /						
/ /						
/ /						
/ /						
/ /						
/ /						
/ /						
/ /						
/ /						
/ /						
/ /						
/ /						
/ /						
/ /						
/ /						
/ /						
/ /						
/ /						
/ /						

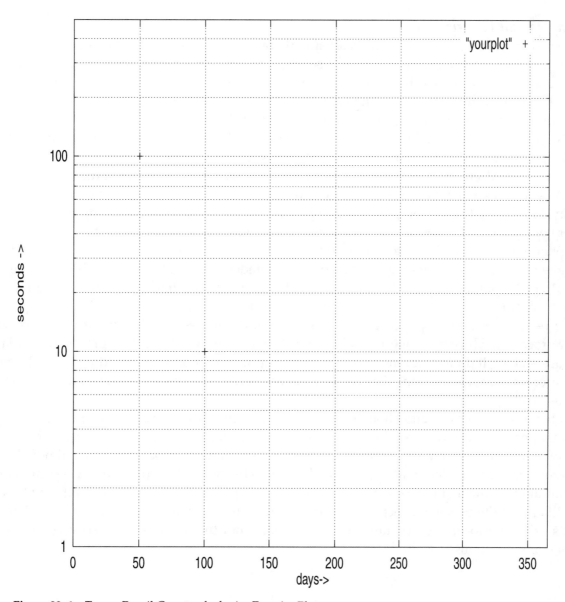

Figure 22–1 Turn a Pencil Counterclockwise Exercise Plot

Discussion

This exercise is a variation on Exercise 11, with a much more difficult turn. Rotating and releasing the pencil is difficult because you must turn your hand in an awkward position. Picking up the pencil is easier than it was in the previous exercise, but releasing it is more difficult because your thumb muscle is already stretched from the turn, and must be stretched more to release the pencil. Opening the hand is always more difficult than is closing it, and now you have to open it in a rotated position, which is even more difficult than it is in a normal position. This exercise is useful because the motion is a part of many aspects of daily living, such as turning a doorknob, turning a faucet on and off, twisting the cap off a bottle, and turning a key in a lock.

Examples and Experiences

I expected this exercise to be very difficult, and it was. I created it as a complement to the previous exercise, so that the two exercises were in a sense symmetric. The inexplicable thing about this exercise is that while it is more difficult to do, it took me less time. How can something more difficult go faster than something that is easier? It may have something to do with the way the pencil is released. As it was difficult to open my hand in a turned position, I threw the pencil out of my hand instead of placing it neatly on the table. After a while, I performed this exercise with great abandon, throwing the pencil as hard as I could, letting gravity work to empty my hand. I developed a clean, swift rotation with my left forearm. (I use this motion now to switch my direction indicator in my car.)

As you can see in Figure 22–2, I progressed nicely for a few months, but experienced a reversal on day 130. On that day I had great trouble picking up the pencil without dropping it. My middle finger bent, pushing the pencil out of my grasp. This made it impossible for me to finish the exercise. This phenomenon actually started around day 100; by day 130, it had become so bad that I decided to change the exercise. I began to use a cardboard cylinder instead of a pencil; it is much larger and easier to pick up. From day 130 to day 300, I used the cardboard cylinder. By day 300 I had regained enough control over my middle finger so that it did not interfere anymore with my grasping, so I used a pencil again. My experience with such a setback indicates that the recovery process is not a linear process in which you continually improve. Instead, another, competing process takes place, in this case making it difficult for me to control the associative motions of my middle finger. If the negative process becomes so strong that you also cannot perform the exercise, you should change exercises as I did.

I have not drawn a straight line in Figure 22–2 because I changed exercises midway through the recovery period. In any case, for the first 100 days there is more or less a straight line, with the beginning of a deviation on day 100. From day 200 on, a straight line can be seen again, although with a different slope. Did another part of my brain become active when I suppressed the negative effect of the neural overflow to my middle finger? Did this other part of my brain have a different time constant? Perhaps the negative effect is still present, but only slows the exercise down. Looking at the results of my performance generates many answers about the nature of the recovery process, but raises many questions as well.

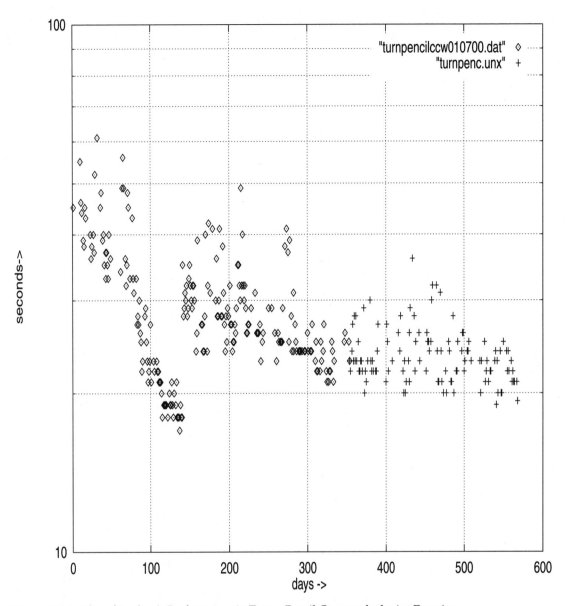

Figure 22–2 Plot of Author's Performance in Turn a Pencil Counterclockwise Exercise

23

Exercise 14: Ten Pencils, Eraser-End First

Purpose: This exercise trains the affected hand to move medium-sized objects (such as pens, pencils, forks, spoons, full drinking glasses, and flowers). The motion is different from the motion used in previous exercises in that you cock your wrist.

Description: In this exercise, you put a pencil in a mug with the tip pointing up. You then take the pencil out, and place it on a table with the tip pointed away from you. You then put the pencil back in the mug with the eraser-end in first. By doing this, you cock your wrist while holding the pencil.

When can you start to do this exercise? You can start to do this exercise when you can pick up a pencil from a mug with your affected hand, and when you can bend your wrist a bit backwards.

What do you need for this exercise? For this exercise you need a thick pen or pencil (thicker than a normal pencil, more like a marker) and a mug. You will also need a stopwatch that can be started, stopped, and restarted.

THE EXERCISE

1. Stand in front of a table on which you have placed the exercise tools.
2. With your unaffected hand, put the pencil in the mug, with the pencil's tip pointing up. Start the stopwatch.
3. With your affected hand, take the pencil out of the mug and place it on the table with the tip pointing away from you.
4. With your affected hand, pick the pencil up, point the tip up by cocking your wrist (this points the tip up in the air), and put the pencil in the mug so that the tip is pointing up again.
5. Repeat steps 3 and 4 a total of 10 times.
6. When you have repeated these steps 10 times, stop the stopwatch.
7. Read the stopwatch time and record it under the "Required Time #1" column in Table 23–1.
8. Repeat steps 3 and 4 and record your time under the "Required Time #2" column in Table 23–1.
9. Repeat steps 3 and 4 for a third time and record your time under the "Required Time #3" column in Table 23–1.

10. Calculate the average of the three required times and record it under the "Average" column in Table 23–1. If you have set a record today, congratulations! Record your score in the column labeled "Records."
11. Plot your average time in Figure 23–1. (See Chapter 9, "How to Record and Plot Your Data," for directions on plotting your data in the graph.)
12. Plot your average time in the "Overall Perspective Plot" in Chapter 36.

Table 23–1   Ten Pencils, Eraser-End First Exercise Table

Date	Day #	Required Time #1	Required Time #2	Required Time #3	Average	Records
/ /						
/ /						
/ /						
/ /						
/ /						
/ /						
/ /						
/ /						
/ /						
/ /						
/ /						
/ /						
/ /						
/ /						
/ /						
/ /						
/ /						
/ /						
/ /						
/ /						
/ /						
/ /						
/ /						
/ /						
/ /						
/ /						
/ /						
/ /						
/ /						

Table 23–1　Ten Pencils, Eraser-End First Exercise Table (*Continued*)

Date	Day #	Required Time #1	Required Time #2	Required Time #3	Average	Records
/ /						
/ /						
/ /						

Discussion

This exercise is similar to Exercise 11, except in this exercise, you bending your wrist upward. This makes it more difficult to hold the pencil. Also, when you put the pencil in the mug you cannot see the mug, because your hand is covering the opening. This makes it difficult to put the pencil in the

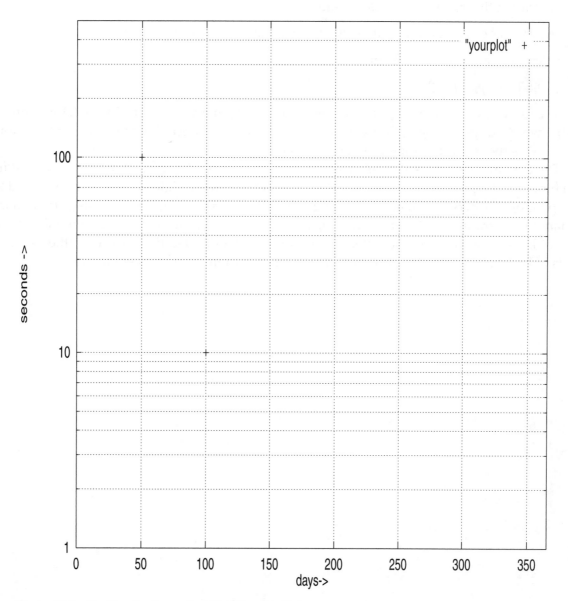

Figure 23–1　Ten Pencils, Eraser-End First Exercise Plot

mug, as you must coordinate your hand with your spatial estimate of where the mug is. This may be difficult for you because the stroke may have wiped out the part of your brain that normally processes such information. Give it a try; you may resuscitate a damaged part of your brain.

Examples and Experiences

I actually began this exercise later than I began many others, so I had experience with the particular hand motion already. This paid off, because the time it took me to do this exercise went down by a time constant of about 66 days. As you can see in Figure 23–2, after around day 200, I did not improve much anymore. Here I reached a plateau, a time I thought was the same as that of a normal person. However, I asked several normal people to do this exercise and found it was difficult to get an average time. The people who did the exercise had many ways of doing it; thus, finding an average was almost useless. My interpretation of Figure 23–2 is as follows: a stroke patient steadily improves for about a year, at which point his or her times are for the most part normal. A mathematical expression describing this recovery process would be:

performance on day x = end value + (beginning value – end value)e $^{-x/timeconstant}$

or, written in a more scientific manner:

$$y(x) = p_e + (p_0 - p_e)e^{-x/\tau}$$

The numbers for beginning value p_0 and end value p_e in my case were 50 and 23. The time constant, τ, was 60 days. Line $y(x)$, the expression of this function, is also drawn in the graph. As you can see, it covers the recovery process reasonably well.

The deviations on days 180, 260, and 360 are not errors in the figure, they are my actual measured times for the exercise. The reason for the deviation is that the night before these days I had taken a sleeping pill. I discovered that the warning printed on sleeping pills, that they can affect your performance in operating machinery or driving a car, is indeed serious. I also discovered that having a night of little or no sleep did not affect my performance. I decided that I would rather have a few nights of bad sleep than a day of impaired performance from taking a sleeping pill.

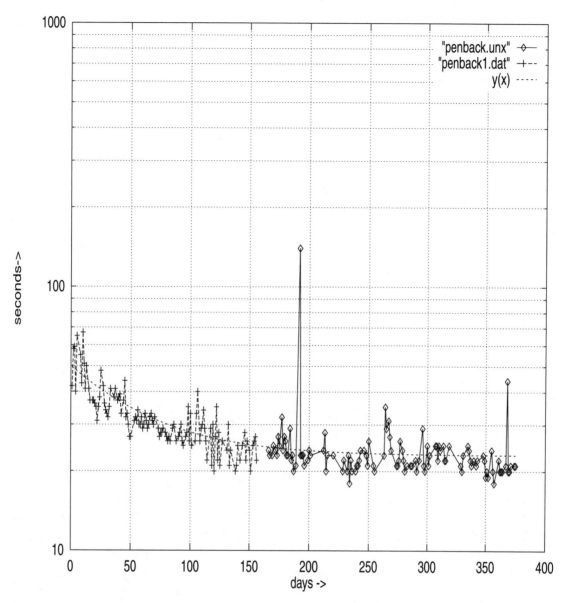

Figure 23–2   Plot of Author's Performance in Ten Pencils, Eraser-End First Exercise

24

Exercise 15: QW

Purpose: This exercise trains the affected hand to use the index finger and middle finger individually.
Description: In this exercise, you touch two neighboring keys on a typewriter or a computer keyboard, one with your index finger, and one with your middle finger. The exercise is named after the first two keys on a keyboard (**Q** and **W**).
When can you start to do this exercise? You can start to do this exercise when you can position your index finger above a key on a typewriter or computer keyboard. (Your middle finger is then automatically roughly above the neighboring key.)
What do you need for this exercise? For this exercise you need a typewriter or computer keyboard. (It does not have to be functional.) If you do not have a keyboard, refer to Appendix III, "Keyboard Layout and Finger Usage," for a diagram of key placement you can use. You will also need a stopwatch that can be started, stopped, and restarted.

THE EXERCISE

1. With your unaffected hand, start the stopwatch.
2. Put your index finger and middle finger on top of the Q and W keys. If your affected hand is your left hand, your index finger will rest on the W key and your middle finger will rest on the Q key. These are the first and second keys on the top row of keys with letters. (The very top row has only numbers and a bunch of other characters.) The W key has two neighbors: to the left is the Q key, to the right is the E key.
3. Press the letter under your index finger with your index finger.
4. Press the letter under your middle finger with your middle finger. You have now pressed a neighboring pair of keys.
5. Move your index finger and middle finger over to the next pair of neighboring keys (that is, the W and E).
6. Press the key under your index finger. (If your affected hand is your left hand, this is the E key; otherwise, it is the W key.)
7. Press the key under your middle finger. (If your affected hand is your left hand, this is the W key; otherwise, it is the E key.)

8. The other neighboring letter pairs on the top row are the E and R, R and T, T and Y, Y and U, U and I. I and O, and O and P keys. Move your index finger and middle finger above each of these pairs and press them, always pressing your index finger first.

9. Move your hand so that your index finger and middle finger are at the first letter pair on the second row (that is, the A and S). Press your index finger on the key underneath it, and then press your middle finger on the key underneath it.

10. The other letter pairs on the middle row are the S and D, D and F, F and G, G and H, H and J, J and K, and K and L keys. Move your index finger and middle finger above each of these pairs and press them, always pressing your index finger first.

11. Move your hand so that your index finger and middle finger are at the beginning of the bottom row, and place them on top of the Z and X keys. Press these keys, using your index finger first.

12. The other letter pairs on the bottom row are the X and C, C and V, V and B, B and N, and N and M keys. Move your index finger and middle finger above each of these pairs and press them, always pressing your index finger first.

13. When you have typed the final N and M key pair, stop the stopwatch with your unaffected hand.

14. Read the stopwatch time and record it under the "Required Time #1" column in Table 24–1.

15. Repeat the entire exercise and record your time under the "Required Time #2" column in Table 24–1.

16. Repeat the entire exercise for a third time and record your time under the "Required Time #3" column in Table 24–1.

17. Calculate the average of the three required times and record it under the "Average" column in Table 24–1. If you have set a record today, congratulations! Record your score in the column labeled "Records."

18. Plot your average time in Figure 24–1. (See Chapter 9, "How to Record and Plot Your Data," for directions on plotting your data in the graph.)

19. Plot your average time in the "Overall Perspective Plot" in Chapter 36.

Table 24–1 QW Exercise Table

Date	Day #	Required Time #1	Required Time #2	Required Time #3	Average	Records
/ /						
/ /						
/ /						
/ /						
/ /						
/ /						
/ /						
/ /						
/ /						
/ /						
/ /						

Table 24–1 QW Exercise Table (*Continued*)

Date	Day #	Required Time #1	Required Time #2	Required Time #3	Average	Records
/ /						
/ /						
/ /						
/ /						
/ /						
/ /						
/ /						
/ /						
/ /						
/ /						
/ /						
/ /						
/ /						
/ /						
/ /						
/ /						
/ /						
/ /						
/ /						
/ /						

Discussion

Although this exercise is not necessarily the easiest or the one you will learn fastest, it may well be the most important exercise in this book. It breaks up the collectivity of the motion of the fingers to ensure that the index finger and the other fingers (in this case, the middle finger) move individually. It also forces the index finger to bend and extend, or to straighten. These motions are of greatest importance and are extremely difficult to do. Because this is such an important exercise, I highly recommend that you perform it on a daily basis.

It is important when doing the exercise that you touch one key with your index finger and the other key with your middle finger. If your thumb, ring finger, or pinky hit a key, don't worry about it. This exercise is not intended to teach you how to type. Instead, it is intended to help you rehabilitate your hand.

You may notice that your index finger wants to bend when your middle finger presses a key. You do not need to be concerned about this "neural overflow," which is brought about when the electrical signal that is meant for your middle finger travels to your index finger as well. Before you touch a new key with your index finger, try to straighten the index finger first. If you cannot straighten it with the proper muscle (the musculus extensor digitorum, which is located on the upper

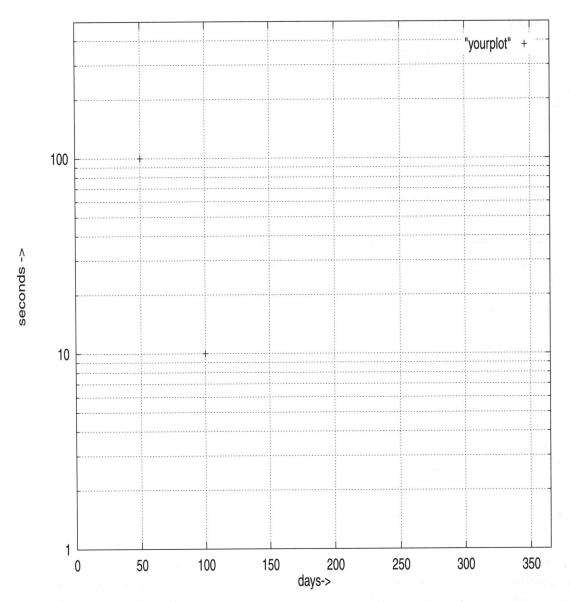

Figure 24–1 QW Exercise Plot

side of your forearm), you may bend it straight with your unaffected hand. However, be careful not to over-stretch it. You may have very little sensation in the joints, and can easily damage them. An alternative way to stretch your fingers is to spread them as wide as you possibly can, thus straightening them. You may also want to rotate your hand while spreading your fingers so that the palm of your hand faces outward. This rotation stretches the muscle that control your index finger. This in turn makes it easier to contract, so a small amount of contraction can have a greater effect.

Don't be surprised if this exercise takes you 5 minutes or more to complete. It is not an easy exercise! It may be a good idea to do this exercise with your unaffected hand first, so you get to know the keyboard a bit. You will also get an idea of how hard you must push on a key to press it down. I don't recommend using a keyboard that is hooked up to a working computer; it will consider your keystrokes as commands. This may in turn distract you from the task at hand: getting your fingers to move.

Examples and Experiences

As you can see in Figure 24–2, the very first time I did this exercise it took me 135 seconds to complete. It took me 11 days to finish it in exactly half that time. Then I entered a period in which I did not improve that quickly anymore. After 120 days, I changed my endurance exercise from 10 minutes on the exercise bike to 1 hour of walking. I had not realized that this was so disastrous until day 200, and even then I did not know that my poor performance was caused by that change. (A full account of these changes is given in Chapter 27, "Exercise 18: FOUR.") Apart from the change in endurance exercise, I saw a daily improvement of around 0.5 percent, or a recovery rate time constant of 197 days (which corresponds to an expected total recovery time of 997 days). If you are faster than I am—congratulations! I am sure you have worked hard at it.

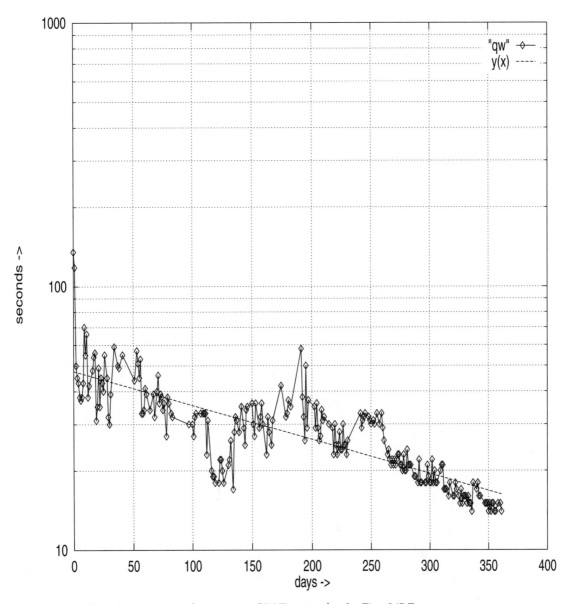

Figure 24–2   Plot of Author's Performance in QW Exercise for the First 365 Days

25

Exercise 16: QWT

Purpose: This exercise trains the affected hand to use the index finger and middle finger individually, and also to activate the thumb.

Description: In this exercise, you touch two neighboring keys on a typewriter or a computer keyboard, one with your index finger, and one with your middle finger. You then touch the spacebar with your thumb. The exercise is named after the first two keys on a keyboard (**Q** and **W**) and the spacebar, which you press with your **Thumb**.

When can you start to do this exercise? You can start to do this exercise when you can position your index finger above a key on a typewriter or computer keyboard. (Your middle finger is then automatically roughly above the neighboring key.) You must also be able to "pronate" your hand. When you pronate your hand, you turn it from a position in which your palm faces down to a position in which your thumb points down.

What do you need for this exercise? For this exercise you need a typewriter or computer keyboard. (It does not have to be functional.) If you do not have a keyboard, refer to Appendix III, "Keyboard Layout and Finger Usage," for a diagram of key placement you can use. You will also need a stopwatch that can be started, stopped, and restarted.

THE EXERCISE

1. With your unaffected hand, start the stopwatch.
2. Put your index finger and middle finger on top of the Q and W keys. If your affected hand is your left hand, your index finger will rest on the W key and your middle finger will rest on the Q key. These are the first and second keys on the top row of keys with letters. (The very top row has only numbers and a bunch of other characters.) The W key has two neighbors: to the left is the Q key, to the right is the E key.
3. Press the letter under your index finger with your index finger.
4. Press the letter under your middle finger with your middle finger. You have now pressed a neighboring pair of keys.
5. Touch your thumb on the spacebar (the long bar closest to you at the bottom of the keyboard). In normal typing the space bar is used to make an empty space between letters.

6. Move your index finger and middle finger over to the next pair of neighboring keys (that is, the W and E).

7. Press the key under your index finger. (If your affected hand is your left hand, this is the E key; otherwise, it is the W key.)

8. Press the key under your middle finger. (If your affected hand is your left hand, this is the W key; otherwise, it is the E key.)

9. Now with your thumb, press the spacebar.

10. The other neighboring letter pairs on the top row are the E and R, R and T, T and Y, Y and U, U and I, I and O, and O and P keys. Move your index finger and middle finger above each of these pairs and press them, always pressing your index finger first. After each pair, press the spacebar with your thumb.

11. Move your hand so that your index finger and middle finger are at the first letter pair on the second row (that is, the A and S). Press your index finger on the key underneath it, and then press your middle finger on the key underneath it. After each pair, press the spacebar with your thumb.

12. The other letter pairs on the middle row are the S and D, D and F, F and G, G and H, H and J, J and K, and K and L keys. Move your index finger and middle finger above each of these pairs and press them, always pressing your index finger first. After each pair, press the spacebar with your thumb.

13. Move your hand so that your index finger and middle finger are at the beginning of the bottom row, and place them on top of the Z and X keys. Press these keys, using your index finger first. Press the spacebar with your thumb.

14. The other letter pairs on the bottom row are the X and C, C and V, V and B, B and N, and N and M keys. Move your index finger and middle finger above each of these pairs and press them, always pressing your index finger first. After each pair, press the spacebar with your thumb.

15. When you have typed the final N and M key pair and spacebar, stop the stopwatch with your unaffected hand.

16. Read the stopwatch time and record it under the "Required Time #1" column in Table 25–1.

17. Repeat the entire exercise and record your time under the "Required Time #2" column in Table 25–1.

18. Repeat the entire exercise for a third time and record your time under the "Required Time #3" column in Table 25–1.

19. Calculate the average of the three required times and record it under the "Average" column in Table 25–1. If you have set a record today, congratulations! Record your score in the column labeled "Records."

20. Plot your average time in Figure 25–1. (See Chapter 9, "How to Record and Plot Your Data," for directions on plotting your data in the graph.)

21. Plot your average time in the "Overall Perspective Plot" in Chapter 36.

Table 25–1 QWT Exercise Table

Date	Day #	Required Time #1	Required Time #2	Required Time #3	Average	Records
/ /						
/ /						
/ /						
/ /						
/ /						
/ /						
/ /						
/ /						
/ /						
/ /						
/ /						
/ /						
/ /						
/ /						
/ /						
/ /						
/ /						
/ /						
/ /						
/ /						
/ /						
/ /						
/ /						
/ /						
/ /						
/ /						
/ /						
/ /						
/ /						
/ /						
/ /						
/ /						

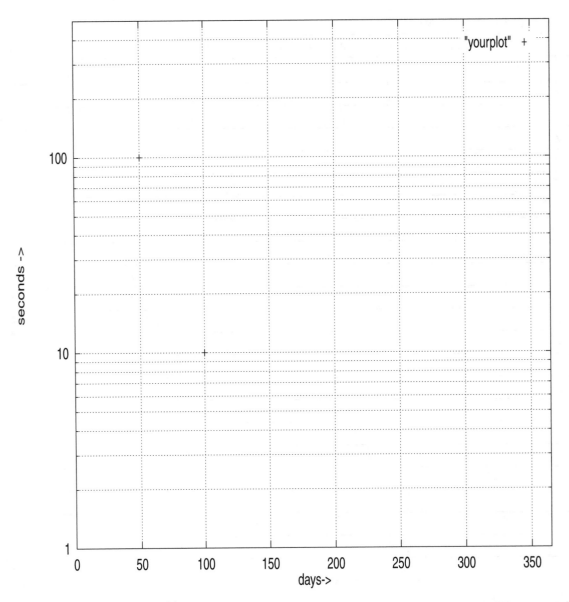

Figure 25–1   QWT Exercise Plot

Discussion

This exercise is a logical extension to Exercise 15. The addition of the thumb motion is important because although you cannot really move your thumb yet, it is a motion you will need in the future.

Examples and Experiences

As you can see in Figure 25–2, after 120 days, I changed my endurance exercise from 10 minutes on the exercise bike to 1 hour of walking. I had not realized that this was so disastrous until day 200, and even then I did not know that my poor performance was caused by that change. (A full account of these changes is given in Chapter 27, "Exercise 18: FOUR.") Due to the changes I made in my exercise in the course of a year, I did not strictly follow the exponential decay curve. In the time period in which I did keep the conditions constant, days 0 to 120 and days 280 to 365, the measurements follow a straight line much more closely. The straight line is the best fitting straight line, it intersects

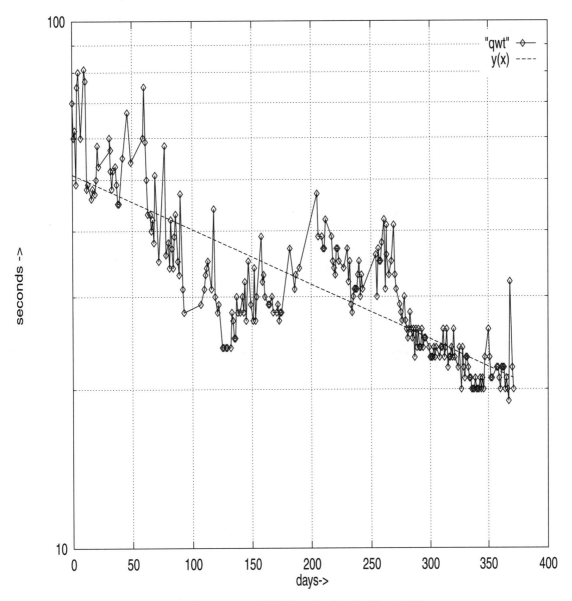

Figure 25–2   Plot of Author's Performance in QWT Exercise for the First 365 Days

the vertical axis at 51 seconds, and it has a slope of -0.00239, which means that the time constant for this exercise is 416 days, or in other words, it took 416 days to reduce the 100 percent disability to 37 percent disability.

26

Exercise 17: THREE

Purpose: This exercise trains the affected hand to use the index finger, middle finger, and ring finger individually.

Description: In this exercise, you touch three neighboring keys on a typewriter or a computer keyboard, one with your index finger, one with your middle finger, and one with your ring finger.

When can you start to do this exercise? You can start to do this exercise when you can position your index finger above a key on a typewriter or computer keyboard. (Your middle finger and ring finger are then automatically roughly above the neighboring keys.)

What do you need for this exercise? For this exercise you need a typewriter or computer keyboard. (It does not have to be functional.) If you do not have a keyboard, refer to Appendix III, "Keyboard Layout and Finger Usage," for a diagram of key placement you can use. You will also need a stopwatch that can be started, stopped, and restarted.

THE EXERCISE

1. With your unaffected hand, start the stopwatch.
2. Put your index finger, middle finger, and ring finger on top of the Q, W, and E keys. If your affected hand is your left hand, your ring finger will rest on the Q key, your middle finger will rest on the W key, and your index finger will rest on the E key. These are the first, second, and third keys on the top row of keys with letters. (The very top row has only numbers and a bunch of other characters.)
3. Press the letter under your index finger with your index finger.
4. Press the letter under your middle finger with your middle finger.
5. Press the letter under your ring finger with your ring finger.
6. Move your index finger, middle finger, and ring finger over to the next set of three neighboring keys (that is, to the W, E, and R keys).
7. Press the key under your index finger. (If your affected hand is your left hand, it is the R key; otherwise, it is the W key.)
8. Press the key under your middle finger (the E key).

9   Press the key under your ring finger. (If your affected hand is your left hand, it is the W key; otherwise, it is the R key.)

10. The other sets of three neighboring keys in the top row are the E, R, and T keys; the R, T, and Y keys; the T, Y, and U keys; the Y, U, and I keys; the U, I, and O keys; and the I, O, and P keys. Move your index finger, middle finger, and ring finger above each of these sets and press them, always pressing your index finger first.

11. Move your hand so that your index finger, middle finger, and ring finger are above the first set of keys in the second row (that is, the A, S, and D keys). Press your index finger on its key, press your middle finger on its the key, then press your ring finger on its key.

12. The remaining sets of three neighboring keys in the middle row are the S, D, and F keys; the D, F, and G keys; the F, G, and H keys; the G, H, and J; the H, J, and K keys; and the J, K, and L keys. Move your index finger, middle finger, ring finger, and pinky above each of these sets and press them, always pressing your index finger first.

13. Move your hand so that your index finger, middle finger, and ring finger are above the first set of keys in the bottom row (that is, the Z, X, and C keys). Press your index finger on its key, press your middle finger on its the key, then press your ring finger on its key.

14. The remaining sets of three neighboring keys in the bottom row are the X, C, and V keys; the C, V, and B keys; the V, B, and N keys; and the B, N, and M keys. Move your index finger, middle finger, ring finger, and pinky above each of these sets and press them, always pressing your index finger first.

15. When you have typed the final B, N, and M key combination, stop the stopwatch with your unaffected hand.

16. Read the stopwatch time and record it under the "Required Time #1" column in Table 26–1.

17. Repeat the entire exercise and record your time under the "Required Time #2" column in Table 26–1.

18. Repeat the entire exercise for a third time and record your time under the "Required Time #3" column in Table 26–1.

19. Calculate the average of the three required times and record it under the "Average" column in Table 26–1. If you have set a record today, congratulations! Record your score in the column labeled "Records."

20. Plot your average time in Figure 26–1. (See Chapter 9, "How to Record and Plot Your Data," for directions on plotting your data in the graph.)

21. Plot your average time in the "Overall Perspective Plot" in Chapter 36.

Table 26–1   THREE Exercise Table

Date	Day #	Required Time #1	Required Time #2	Required Time #3	Average	Records
/ /						
/ /						
/ /						
/ /						
/ /						
/ /						
/ /						

Table 26–1   THREE Exercise Table (*Continued*)

Date	Day #	Required Time #1	Required Time #2	Required Time #3	Average	Records
/ /						
/ /						
/ /						
/ /						
/ /						
/ /						
/ /						
/ /						
/ /						
/ /						
/ /						
/ /						
/ /						
/ /						
/ /						
/ /						
/ /						
/ /						
/ /						
/ /						
/ /						
/ /						
/ /						

Discussion

This exercise is another logical extension to Exercise 15. The additional motion of your ring finger comes rather naturally, therefore the exercise is not that much harder than Exercise 15.

> *A woman who was much given to chit-chat,*
> *had once given birth to a triplet.*
> *But once she was "struck,"*
> *by major bad luck,*
> *She said "Three?, No forget it, I did that!"*

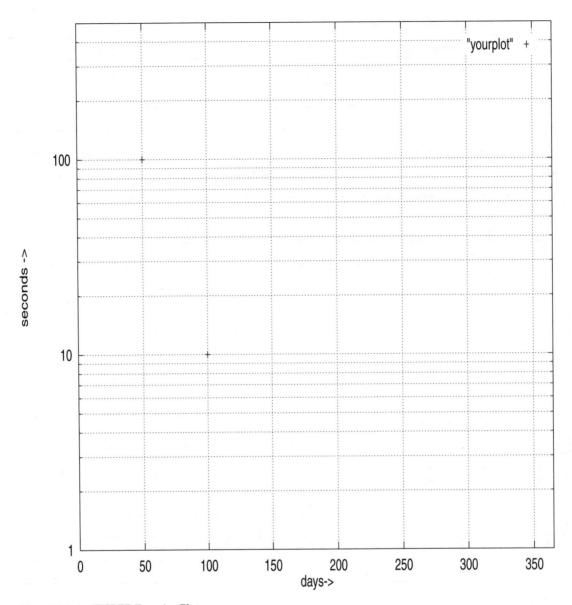

Figure 26–1   THREE Exercise Plot

Examples and Experiences

I have plotted the times it took me to do this exercise for the first 450 days in Figure 26–2.

In Figure 26–3 I have presented the same data only in the format of a logarithmic plot. Notice that points near the upper part of the graph are now further apart, while the lower part is more evenly spread out. Also notice that the plot can be more or less represented by a straight line. The best fitting straight line has also been drawn.

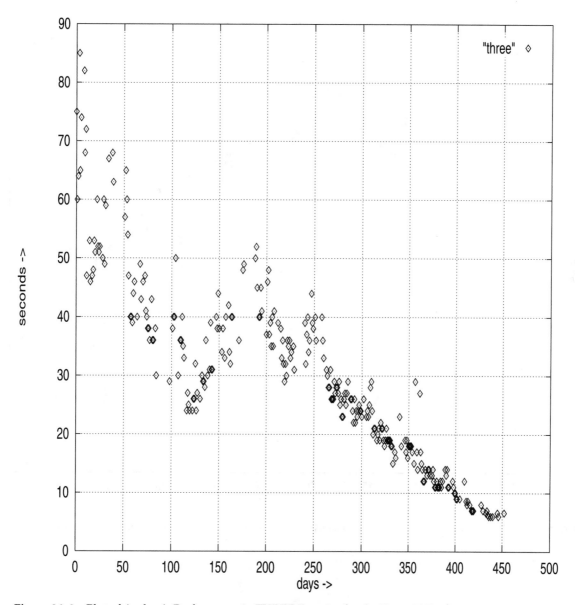

Figure 26–2   Plot of Author's Performance in THREE Exercise for the First 450 Days

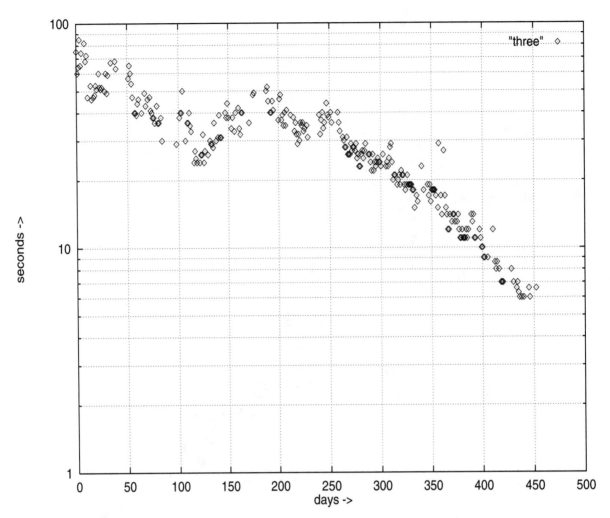

Figure 26–3   Plot of Author's Performance in THREE Exercise for the First 450 Days on a Logarithmic Plot

27

Exercise 18: FOUR

Purpose: This exercise trains the affected hand to use the index finger, middle finger, ring finger, and pinky individually.

Description: In this exercise, you touch four neighboring keys on a typewriter or a computer keyboard, one with your index finger, one with your middle finger, one with your ring finger, and one with your pinky.

When can you start to do this exercise? You can start to do this exercise when you can position your index finger above a key on a typewriter or computer keyboard. (Your middle finger, ring finger, and pinky are then automatically roughly above the neighboring keys.) You can start this exercise on the same day as you started Exercise 15, or you can wait a couple of days.

What do you need for this exercise? For this exercise you need a typewriter or computer keyboard. (It does not have to be functional.) If you do not have a keyboard, refer to Appendix III, "Keyboard Layout and Finger Usage," for a diagram of key placement you can use. You will also need a stopwatch that can be started, stopped, and restarted.

THE EXERCISE

1. With your unaffected hand, start the stopwatch.
2. Put your index finger, middle finger, ring finger, and pinky on top of the Q, W, E, and R keys. If your affected hand is your left hand, your pinky will rest on the Q key, your ring finger will rest on the W key, your middle finger will rest on the E key, your index finger will rest on the R key. These are the first, second, third, and fourth keys on the top row of keys with letters. (The very top row has only numbers and a bunch of other characters.)
3. Press the letter under your index finger with your index finger.
4. Press the letter under your middle finger with your middle finger.
5. Press the letter under your ring finger with your ring finger.
6. Press the letter under your pinky with your pinky.
7. Move your index finger, middle finger, ring finger, and pinky over to the next set of four neighboring keys (that is, to the W, E, R, and T keys).

8. Press the key under your index finger. (If your affected hand is your left hand, it is the T key; otherwise, it is the W key.)
9. Press the key under your middle finger (the E or R key).
10 Press the key under your ring finger (the E or R key).
11. Press the key under your pinky. (If your affected hand is your left hand, it is the W key; otherwise, it is the T key.)
12. The other sets of four neighboring keys on the top row are the E, R, T, and Y keys; the R, T, Y, and U keys; the T, Y, U, and I keys; the Y, U, I, and O keys; and the U, I, O, and P keys. Move your index finger, middle finger, ring finger, and pinky above each of these sets and press them, always pressing your index finger first.
13. Move your hand so that your index finger, middle finger, ring finger, and pinky are above the first set of keys in the second row (that is, the A, S, D, and F keys). Press your index finger on its key, press your middle finger on its the key, press your ring finger on its key, then press your pinky on its key.
14. The remaining sets of four neighboring keys in the middle row are the S, D, F, and G keys; the D, F, G, and H keys; the F, G, H, and J keys; the G, H, J, and K keys; and the H, J, K, and L keys. Move your index finger, middle finger, ring finger, and pinky above each of these sets and press them, always pressing your index finger first.
15. Move your fingers now to the beginning of the bottom row, and place them above the Z, X, C, and V keys. Press your index finger on its key, press your middle finger on its the key, press your ring finger on its key, then press your pinky on its key.
16. The remaining sets of four neighboring keys in the bottom row are the X, C, V, and B keys; the C, V, B, and N keys; and the V, B, N, and M keys. Move your index finger, middle finger, ring finger, and pinky above each of these sets and press them, always pressing your index finger first.
17. When you have typed the final V, B, N, and M key combination, stop the stopwatch with your unaffected hand.
18. Read the stopwatch time and record it under the "Required Time #1" column in Table 27–1.
19. Repeat the entire exercise and record your time under the "Required Time #2" column in Table 27–1.
20. Repeat the entire exercise for a third time and record your time under the "Required Time #3" column in Table 27–1.
21. Calculate the average of the three required times and record it under the "Average" column in Table 27–1. If you have set a record today, congratulations! Record your score in the column labeled "Records."
22. Plot your average time in Figure 27–1. (See Chapter 9, "How to Record and Plot Your Data," for directions on plotting your data in the graph.)
23. Plot your average time in the "Overall Perspective Plot" in Chapter 36.

Table 27–1 FOUR Exercise Table

Date	Day #	Required Time #1	Required Time #2	Required Time #3	Average	Records
/ /						
/ /						
/ /						
/ /						
/ /						
/ /						
/ /						
/ /						
/ /						
/ /						
/ /						
/ /						
/ /						
/ /						
/ /						
/ /						
/ /						
/ /						
/ /						
/ /						
/ /						
/ /						
/ /						
/ /						
/ /						
/ /						
/ /						
/ /						
/ /						
/ /						

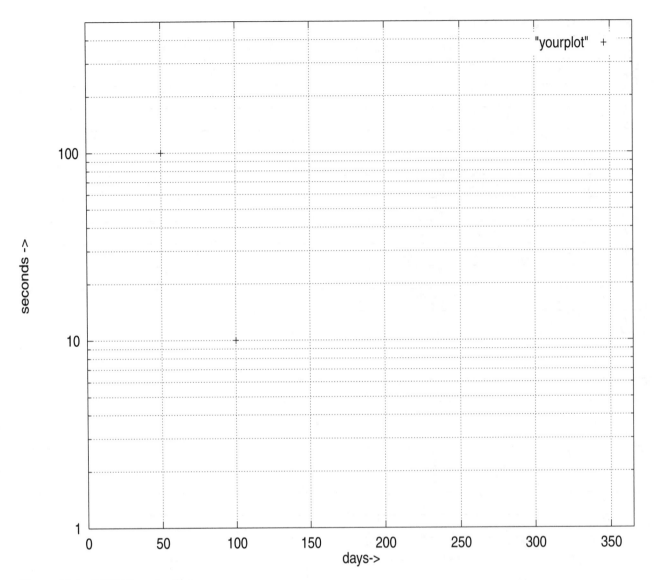

Figure 27–1 FOUR Exercise Plot

Discussion

This exercise is another logical extension to Exercise 15. The addition of the pinky motion is quite simple, although as with all exercises in this book, the exercise is very challenging.

Examples and Experiences

I have plotted the times it took me to do this exercise for the first 450 days in Figure 27–2.

In Figure 27–3 I have presented the same data only in the format of a logarithmic plot. As you can see, after 120 days, I changed my endurance exercise from 10 minutes on the exercise bike to 1 hour of walking. I had not realized that this was so disastrous until day 200, and even then I did not know that my poor performance was caused by that change. Due to the changes I made in my exercise in the course of a year, I did not strictly follow the exponential decay curve. My time constant for this period was around 100 days. During days 250 though 450 I had returned to the biking

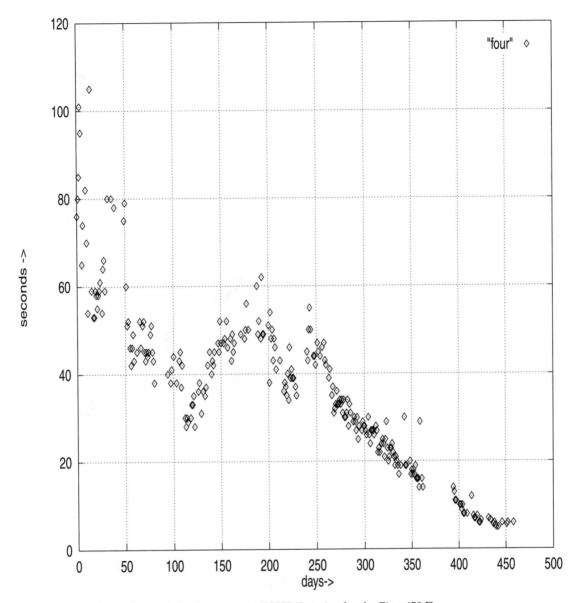

Figure 27–2   Plot of Author's Performance in FOUR Exercise for the First 450 Days

exercise, and my old time constant shows up again (actually it is slightly shorter, 90 days, because from days 250 to 450 I did the exercise three times per day, while from day 0 to 120, I did it only once per day).

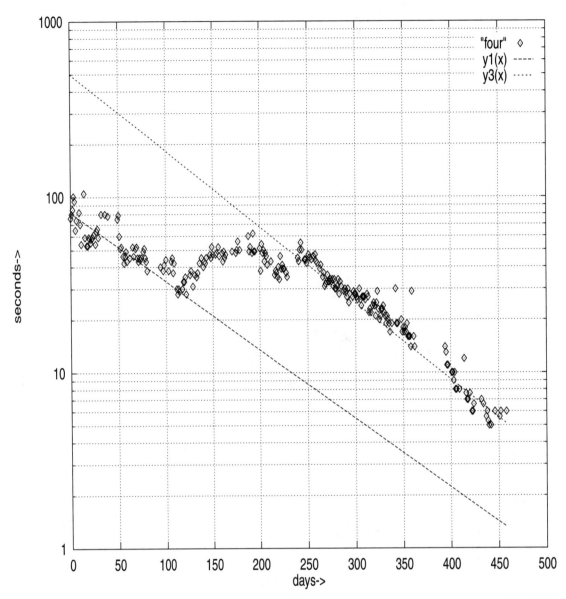

Figure 27–3   Plot of Author's Performance in FOUR Exercise for the First 450 Days on a Logarithmic Plot

28

Exercise 19: FIVE

Purpose: The purpose of this exercise is to train the affected hand to use the index, middle finger, ring finger, and little finger individually, as well as to integrate a motion with the thumb.

Description: In this exercise, you touch four neighboring keys on a typewriter or a computer keyboard, one with your index finger, one with your middle finger, one with your ring finger, and one with your pinky. You then touch the spacebar with your thumb.

When can you start to do this exercise? You can start to do this exercise when you can position your index finger above a key on a typewriter or computer keyboard. (Your middle finger, ring finger, and pinky are then automatically roughly above the neighboring keys.) You can start this exercise on the same day as you started Exercise 15, or you can wait a couple of days.

What do you need for this exercise? For this exercise you need a typewriter or computer keyboard. (It does not have to be functional.) If you do not have a keyboard, refer to Appendix III, "Keyboard Layout and Finger Usage," for a diagram of key placement you can use. You will also need a stopwatch that can be started, stopped, and restarted.

THE EXERCISE

1. With your unaffected hand, start the stopwatch.
2. Put your index finger, middle finger, ring finger, and pinky on top of the Q, W, E, and R keys. If your affected hand is your left hand, your pinky will rest on the Q key, your ring finger will rest on the W key, your middle finger will rest on the E key, your index finger will rest on the R key. These are the first, second, third, and fourth keys on the top row of keys with letters. (The very top row has only numbers and a bunch of other characters.)
3. Press the letter under your index finger with your index finger.
4. Press the letter under your middle finger with your middle finger.
5. Press the letter under your ring finger with your ring finger.
6. Press the letter under your pinky with your pinky.
7. Now touch the spacebar with your thumb.
8. Move your index finger, middle finger, ring finger, and pinky over to the next set of four neighboring keys (that is, to the W, E, R, and T keys).

9. Press the key under your index finger. (If your affected hand is your left hand, it is the T key; otherwise, it is the W key.)
10. Press the key under your middle finger (the E or R key).
11. Press the key under your ring finger (the E or R key).
12. Press the key under your pinky. (If your affected hand is your left hand, it is the W key; otherwise, it is the T key.)
13. Touch the spacebar with your thumb.
14. The other sets of four neighboring keys on the top row are the E, R, T, and Y keys; the R, T, Y, and U keys; the T, Y, U, and I keys; the Y, U, I, and O keys; and the U, I, O, and P keys. Move your index finger, middle finger, ring finger, and pinky above each of these sets and press them, always pressing your index finger first. Then press the spacebar with your thumb.
15. Move your hand so that your index finger, middle finger, ring finger, and pinky are above the first set of keys in the second row (that is, the A, S, D, and F keys). Press your index finger on its key, press your middle finger on its the key, press your ring finger on its key, then press your pinky on its key. Then press the spacebar with your thumb.
16. The remaining sets of four neighboring keys in the middle row are the S, D, F, and G keys; the D, F, G, and H keys; the F, G, H, and J keys; the G, H, J, and K keys; and the H, J, K, and L keys. Move your index finger, middle finger, ring finger, and pinky above each of these sets and press them, always pressing your index finger first. Then press the spacebar with your thumb.
17. Move your fingers now to the beginning of the bottom row, and place them above the Z, X, C, and V keys. Press your index finger on its key, press your middle finger on its the key, press your ring finger on its key, then press your pinky on its key. Then press the spacebar with your thumb.
18. The remaining sets of four neighboring keys in the bottom row are the X, C, V, and B keys; the C, V, B, and N keys; and the V, B, N, and M keys. Move your index finger, middle finger, ring finger, and pinky above each of these sets and press them, always pressing your index finger first. Then press the spacebar with your thumb.
19. When you have typed the final V, B, N, and M key combination, stop the stopwatch with your unaffected hand.
20. Read the stopwatch time and record it under the "Required Time #1" column in Table 28–1.
21. Repeat the entire exercise and record your time under the "Required Time #2" column in Table 28–1.
22. Repeat the entire exercise for a third time and record your time under the "Required Time #3" column in Table 28–1.
23. Calculate the average of the three required times and record it under the "Average" column in Table 28–1. If you have set a record today, congratulations! Record your score in the column labeled "Records."
24. Plot your average time in Figure 28–1. (See Chapter 9, "How to Record and Plot Your Data," for directions on plotting your data in the graph.)
25. Plot your average time in the "Overall Perspective Plot" in Chapter 36.

Table 28–1   FIVE Exercise Table

Date	Day #	Required Time #1	Required Time #2	Required Time #3	Average	Records
/ /						
/ /						
/ /						
/ /						
/ /						
/ /						
/ /						
/ /						
/ /						
/ /						
/ /						
/ /						
/ /						
/ /						
/ /						
/ /						
/ /						
/ /						
/ /						
/ /						
/ /						
/ /						
/ /						
/ /						
/ /						
/ /						
/ /						
/ /						
/ /						
/ /						
/ /						

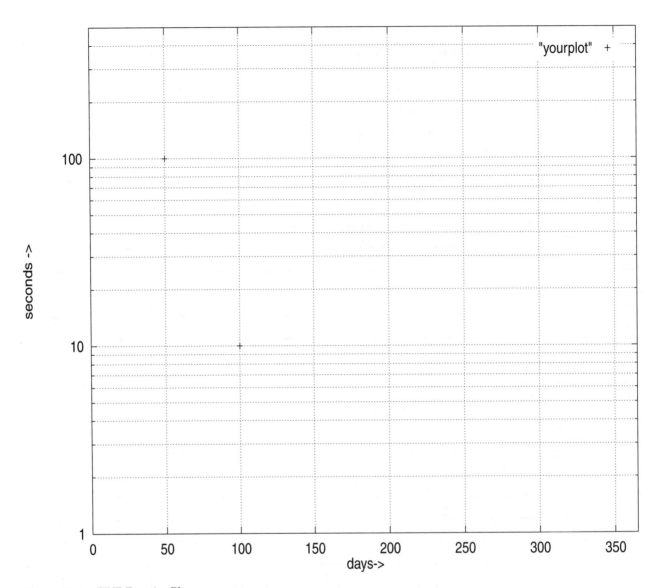

Figure 28–1   FIVE Exercise Plot

Discussion

This exercise is another logical extension to Exercise 15. The additional thumb motion makes this a complete exercise, integrating the motions of the fingers with the motion of the thumb. This is also not an easy exercise. All exercises in this book are difficult for stroke survivors, so don't feel bad if it takes you a while to get the hang of it.

Examples and Experiences

I have plotted the times it took me to do this exercise for the first 450 days in Figure 28–2. Also given in this plot is the best fitting exponential decay curve. Notice that the first three times I did this exercise, it took me 80, 85, and 101 seconds to complete it.

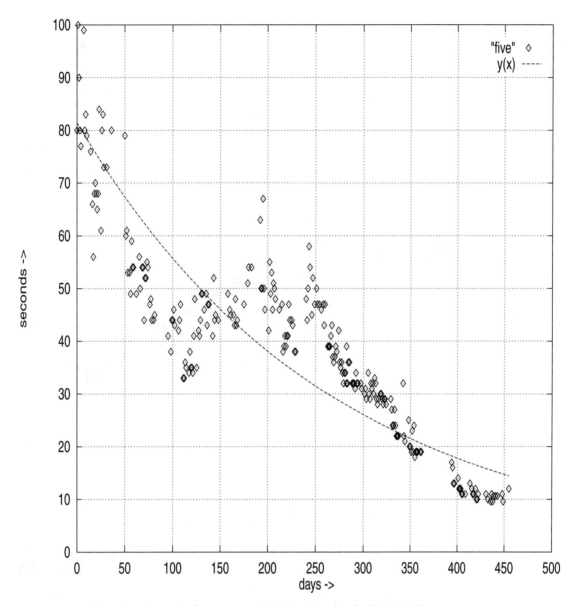

Figure 28–2   Plot of Author's Performance in FIVE Exercise for the First 450 Days

In Figure 28–3 I have plotted the same times but on a logarithmic scale. I have also drawn the best fitting straight lines for the first 120 days of the exercise and for the last days of the exercise. As you can see, the behavior of these measurements follows an exponential decay function perfectly, as the measurements are almost precisely on the straight line.

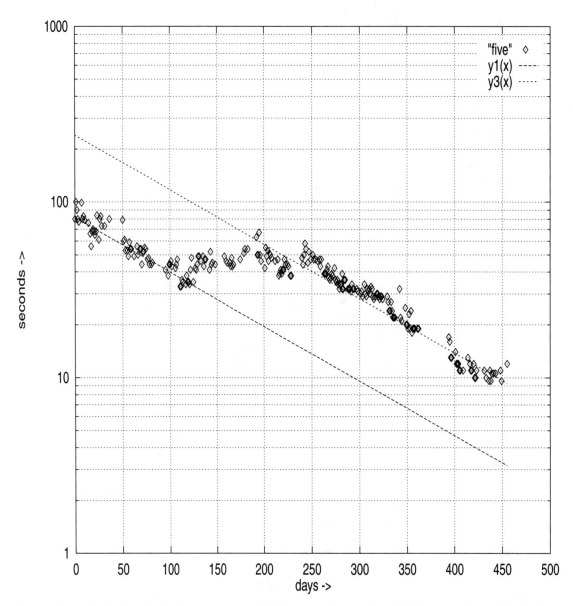

Figure 28–3   Plot of Author's Performance in FIVE Exercise for the First 450 Days on a Logarithmic Plot

29

Exercise 20: WAFERS10/MONOPOLY10

Purpose: The purpose of this exercise is to train the affected hand to use the fingers individually.

Description: In this exercise, you type 10 times the word "wafers" with the left hand or the word "monopoly" with the right hand (depending on which hand is your affected hand). First the word is typed, then the number of times it was typed, so that the typed word looks like: WAFERS1, WAFERS2, WAFERS3, WAFERS4, and so on (or MONOPOLY1, MONOPOLY2, MONOPOLY3, MONOPOLY4, and so on). By typing the number after the word you avoid getting confused over how many times you have typed it. Also, you type more words, and your time measurement is therefore more accurate.

When can you start to do this exercise? You can start to do this exercise when you have done Exercise 19, "FIVE" for a week.

What do you need for this exercise? For this exercise you need a typewriter or computer keyboard. (It does not have to be functional.) If you do not have a keyboard, refer to Appendix III, "Keyboard Layout and Finger Usage," for a diagram of key placement you can use. You will also need a stopwatch that can be started, stopped, and restarted.

THE EXERCISE

If your affected hand is your left hand:

1. With your unaffected hand, start the stopwatch.
2. Put your **ring** finger on the W and press the key.
3. Put your **little** finger on the A and press the key.
4. Put your **index** finger on the F and press the key.
5. Put your **middle** finger on the E and press the key.
6. Put your **index** finger on the R and press the key.
7. Put your **ring** finger on the S and press the key.
8. Put your **index** finger on the number 1 and press the key.
9. Type the word WAFERS in the same way but now finish it off by typing the number 2 with your **index** finger. Repeat this process until you reach WAFERS10 (typing both the 1 and the 0 with your **index** finger).

10. Stop the stopwatch with your unaffected hand.
11. Read the stopwatch time and record it under the "Required Time #1" column in Table 29–1.
12. Repeat the entire exercise and record your time under the "Required Time #2" column in Table 29–1.
13. Repeat the entire exercise for a third time and record your time under the "Required Time #3" column in Table 29–1.
14. Calculate the average of the three required times and record it under the "Average" column in Table 29–1. If you have set a record today, congratulations! Record your score in the column labeled "Records."
15. Plot your average time in Figure 29–1. (See Chapter 9, "How to Record and Plot Your Data," for directions on plotting your data in the graph.)
16. Plot your average time in the "Overall Perspective Plot" in Chapter 36.

If your affected hand is your right hand:

1. With your unaffected hand, start the stopwatch.
2. Put your **index** finger on the M and press the key.
3. Put your **ring** finger on the O and press the key.
4. Put your **index** finger on the N and press the key.
5. Put your **ring** finger on the O and press the key.
6. Put your **little** finger on the P and press the key.
7. Put your **ring** finger on the O and press the key.
8. Put your **ring** finger on the L and press the key.
9. Put your **index** finger on the Y and press the key.
10. Put your **index** finger on the number 1 and press the key.
11. Type the word MONOPOLY in the same way but now finish it off by typing the number 2 with your **index** finger. Repeat this process until you reach MONOPOLY10 (typing both the 1 and the 0 with your **index** finger).
12. Follow steps 10 through 16 as indicated for left-hand use.

Table 29–1   WAFERS10/MONOPOLY10 Exercise Table

Date	Day #	Required Time #1	Required Time #2	Required Time #3	Average	Records
/ /						
/ /						
/ /						
/ /						
/ /						
/ /						
/ /						
/ /						
/ /						
/ /						

Table 29–1   WAFERS10/MONOPOLY10 Exercise Table (*Continued*)

Date	Day #	Required Time #1	Required Time #2	Required Time #3	Average	Records
/ /						
/ /						
/ /						
/ /						
/ /						
/ /						
/ /						
/ /						
/ /						
/ /						
/ /						
/ /						
/ /						
/ /						
/ /						
/ /						
/ /						
/ /						
/ /						
/ /						
/ /						

Discussion

This exercise may be the second most important exercise in this book, after Exercise 15. Please note that you may change the word if you like. If you have a military background, you may prefer to type the word "warfare" instead of "wafers." If you like fashion you may prefer to type the word "street-dress"; if you are a computer person you may prefer to type the word "inputoutput." You may come up with any word that is typed exclusively with one hand. You may even change "monopoly" into "polonium" for the right-hand exercise if you really want. (Polonium is an element in the trans-uranium series. It does not occur naturally, but is a by-product of some nuclear reactions.)

Even if your right hand is your affected hand, you may type "wafers" if you would prefer that over "monopoly"; it all depends on your preference. There are not all that many words with enough letters (at least six) that you can type with the right hand only (that is, with the keys to the right of the letters Y in the top row, H in the middle row, and B in the bottom row). At least, I could not come up with more than the ones I mentioned. (If you find an interesting word, please write it on a postcard and send it to the address of the publisher, who can forward it to me for inclusion in a possible second printing of this book. You will be dutifully acknowledged.)

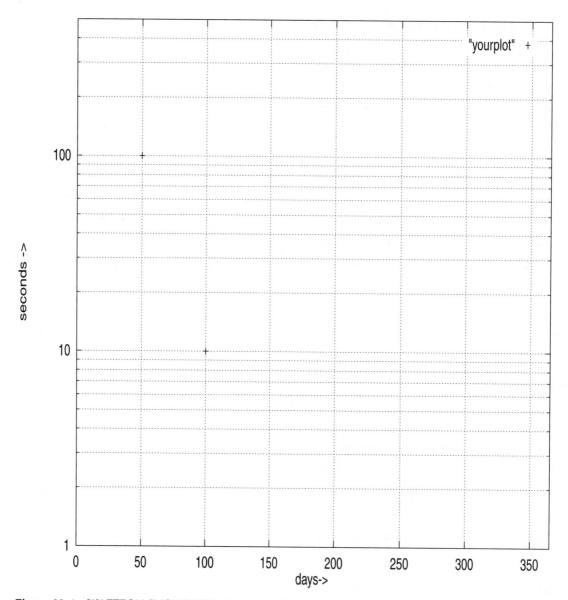

Figure 29–1   WAFERS10/MONOPOLY10 Exercise Plot

Examples and Experiences

Since I am an Associate Professor of Electrical Engineering in the field of silicon processing, which uses thin slices of material called "wafers," I had to type the word wafers numerous times before I had a stroke. It struck me many years ago that this word was typed with the left hand only. So when I had to retrain my hand, I thought it was a good idea to use that word as a training tool. Since this is a rather complex exercise involving all fingers, the initial phase of learning is rather short.

After 258 days of exercising, I suddenly noticed that the rhythm of my motions had changed in this exercise. Until then, I had pressed each key individually. Then I noticed that instead of the familiar rhythm of boom—boom—boom—boom—boom—boom, it had changed to boom—boom—boomboom—boom—boom. The third and fourth key had more or less merged. When I looked a little closer at what I was doing, I saw that those keys were the F and E. The F was pressed with the index finger and the E was pressed with the middle finger. This sequence of index and middle finger was precisely the movement that was used in Exercise 15, "QW." The two-finger "QW" exercise had helped me improve my typing speed when I did the multi-finger exercise of typing the word "wafers."

On day 272, I noticed that the rhythm had changed again. Now I found that it was boomboom—boomboom—boom—boom. The first and second key had also merged. When I looked a little closer at what I was doing, I realized that the W and A were being pressed by my ring finger and little finger. This sequence was a part of the "FOUR" and "FIVE" exercises (Exercises 18 and 19) in which the ring finger and little finger are used successively. Here was proof that the training of individual elemental motions had resulted in the integration of these motions in a larger pattern. The time it took for this to happen was another surprise: 258 or 272 days was just a little longer than the recovery rate constant for the "QW" and "FOUR" exercises when I had measured those for the very first time (which were 197 and 202 days, respectively). This brought me to make the following assumption: After a time period equal to a recovery rate constant, the motion of an exercise can become an integral part of a more complex pattern when that pattern is also an exercise.

There are three straight lines in Figure 29–2: y1(x), y2(x) and y3(x). The first line is the best-fitting straight line for the first 120 days; it has a recovery rate time constant of 133 days. The next line is the best-fitting straight line for the last 120 days; it has a time constant of 148 days. The third line is the best-fitting line for all 365 days; this one has a time constant of 329 days. As you see, the last straight line is pretty useless; it does not follow the measured points because I did not keep all conditions constant during the 365 days. (The conditions of exercising during the first 120 days were the same as those for the last 120 days; the time constants are also pretty much the same, and they are probably the right value for this exercise.)

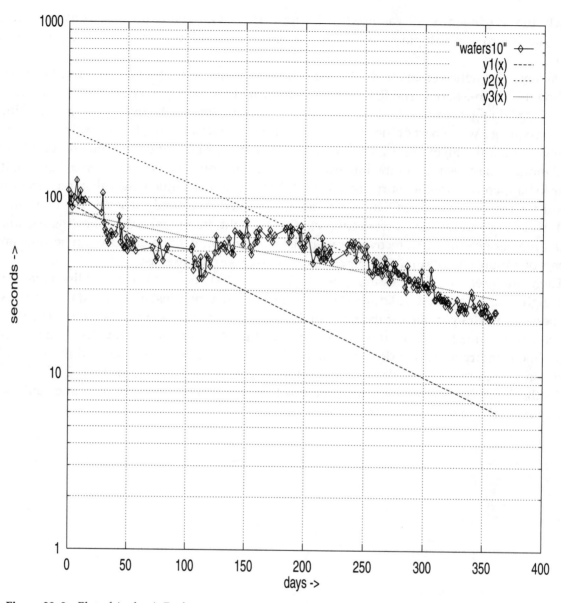

Figure 29–2   Plot of Author's Performance in WAFERS10 Exercise for the First 365 Days

30

Exercise 21: The Quick Fox

Purpose: This exercise trains the affected hand to use all fingers individually, and to integrate their motions with those of the fingers of the unaffected hand.

Description: In this exercise, you type with both hands the sentence "the quick brown fox jumps over the lazy dog."

When can you start to do this exercise? You can start to do this exercise when you have done Exercise 20 for a week.

What do you need for this exercise? For this exercise you need a typewriter or computer keyboard. (It does not have to be functional.) If you do not have a keyboard, refer to Appendix III, "Keyboard Layout and Finger Usage," for a diagram of key placement you can use. You will also need a stopwatch that can be started, stopped, and restarted.

THE EXERCISE

Sit down in front of the keyboard with this book and the stopwatch on your unaffected side. Put your unaffected hand on your knee before you start, and make sure that it is relaxed. Relax your shoulders and take a deep breath.

1. With your unaffected hand, start the stopwatch.
2. With both hands, type the sentence "the quick brown fox jumps over the lazy dog" using the appropriate finger for each key. Use the thumb of your unaffected hand for the spacebar.
3. When you are done, stop the stopwatch with your unaffected hand.
4. Read the stopwatch time and record it under the "Required Time #1" column in Table 30–1.
5. Repeat the entire exercise and record your time under the "Required Time #2" column in Table 30–1.
6. Repeat the entire exercise for a third time and record your time under the "Required Time #3" column in Table 30–1.
7. Calculate the average of the three required times and record it under the "Average" column in Table 30–1. If you have set a record today, congratulations! Record your score in the column labeled "Records."

8. Plot your average time in Figure 30–1. (See Chapter 9, "How to Record and Plot Your Data," for directions on plotting your data in the graph.)
9. Plot your average time in the "Overall Perspective Plot" in Chapter 36.

Table 30–1   The Quick Fox Exercise Table

Date	Day #	Required Time #1	Required Time #2	Required Time #3	Average	Records
/ /						
/ /						
/ /						
/ /						
/ /						
/ /						
/ /						
/ /						
/ /						
/ /						
/ /						
/ /						
/ /						
/ /						
/ /						
/ /						
/ /						
/ /						
/ /						
/ /						
/ /						
/ /						
/ /						
/ /						
/ /						
/ /						
/ /						
/ /						
/ /						
/ /						

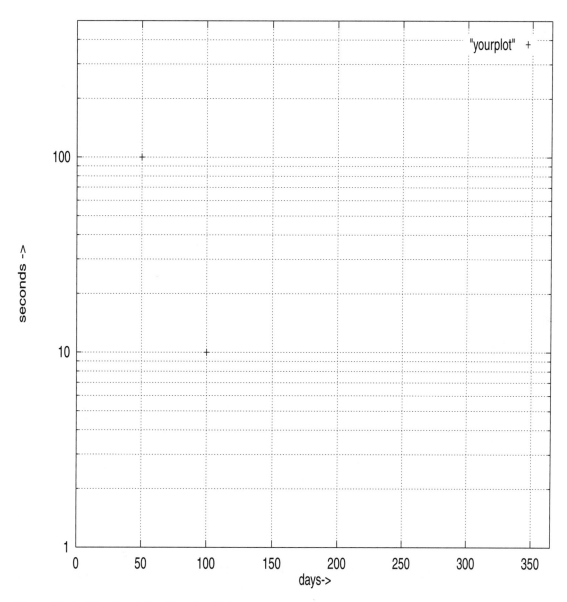

Figure 30–1 The Quick Fox Exercise Plot

Discussion

In general, this exercise gets both hands working together. Although there are some unexpected difficulties, this is a surprisingly easy exercise. The sequence of the letters A and Z in the word "lazy" is typed with the little finger only, which is a bit difficult if your affected hand is your left hand.

Examples and Experiences

In Figure 30–2 I have plotted my times for this exercise. Notice that I needed around 20 seconds for this sentence in the beginning and that it took me more than 9 months to get this time down to 14 seconds. This means that the recovery rate constant is almost 1 year. Also notice that the measurements are relatively smooth, and that there is not a lot of scattering. Problems associated with learning by random trial and error are not present in this exercise.

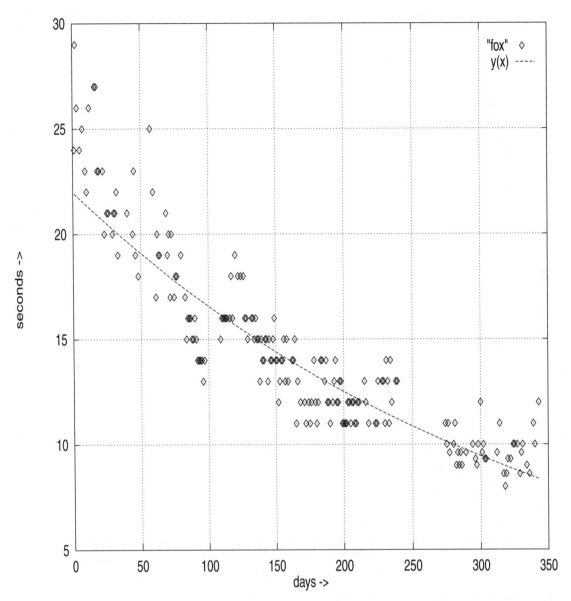

Figure 30–2   Plot of Author's Performance in The Quick Fox Exercise for the First 365 Days

In Figure 30–3 you see the same data displayed in a logarithmic plot. The times follow the dotted line remarkably well. The time constant for this exercise was 355 days.

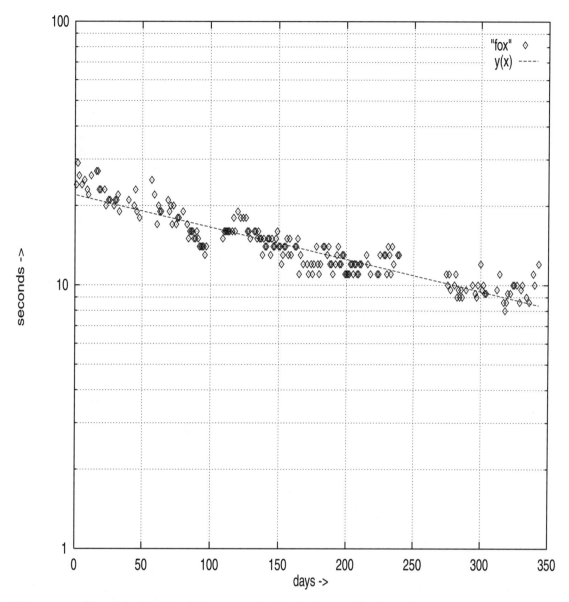

Figure 30–3 Plot of Author's Performance in The Quick Fox Exercise for the First 365 Days in a Logarithmic Plot

31

Exercise 22: Racecar

Purpose: This exercise trains the affected hand to use all the fingers individually by typing a long sentence. The sequence of the finger movements is different and more complex than in the previous exercises.

Description: In this exercise, you type a sentence with your affected hand only. The exercise is named after the palindrome (a word that reads the same forwards and backwards) that occurs in the sentence.

When can you start to do this exercise? You can start to do this exercise when you have done "Quick Fox" for a week.

What do you need for this exercise? For this exercise you need a typewriter or computer keyboard. (It does not have to be functional.) If you do not have a keyboard, refer to Appendix III, "Keyboard Layout and Finger Usage," for a diagram of key placement you can use. You will also need a stopwatch that can be started, stopped, and restarted.

THE EXERCISE

1. With your unaffected hand, start the stopwatch.
2. With your affected hand, type the sentence "we were raw scarred racers, we raced sacred racecars fastest."
3. When you are done, stop the stopwatch with your unaffected hand.
4. Read the stopwatch time and record it under the "Required Time #1" column in Table 31–1.
5. Repeat the entire exercise and record your time under the "Required Time #2" column in Table 31–1.
6. Repeat the entire exercise for a third time and record your time under the "Required Time #3" column in Table 31–1.
7. Calculate the average of the three required times and record it under the "Average" column in Table 31–1. If you have set a record today, congratulations! Record your score in the column labeled "Records."
8. Plot your average time in Figure 31–1, marking your time with a cross (+). (See Chapter 9, "How to Record and Plot Your Data," for directions on plotting your data in the graph.)

9. Plot your average time in the "Overall Perspective Plot" in Chapter 36.

10. Now complete the exercise with the sentence: "we ex-stars wear streetdresses at crazy catered feasts." (You don't have to type the hyphen.)

11. When you are done, stop the stopwatch with your unaffected hand.

12. Read the stopwatch time and record it under the "Required Time #1" column in Table 31–2.

13. Repeat the entire exercise and record your time under the "Required Time #2" column in Table 31–2.

14. Repeat the entire exercise for a third time and record your time under the "Required Time #3" column in Table 31–2.

15. Calculate the average of the three required times and record it under the "Average" column in Table 31–1. If you have set a record today, congratulations! Record your score in the column labeled "Records."

16. Plot your average time in Figure 31–1, marking your time with a diamond. (See Chapter 9, "How to Record and Plot Your Data," for directions on plotting your data in the graph.)

17. Plot your average time in the "Overall Perspective Plot" in Chapter 36.

Table 31–1   Racecar Exercise 1 Table

Date	Day #	Required Time #1	Required Time #2	Required Time #3	Average	Records
/ /						
/ /						
/ /						
/ /						
/ /						
/ /						
/ /						
/ /						
/ /						
/ /						
/ /						
/ /						
/ /						
/ /						
/ /						
/ /						
/ /						
/ /						
/ /						
/ /						
/ /						

Table 31–1   Racecar Exercise 1 Table (*Continued*)

Date	Day #	Required Time #1	Required Time #2	Required Time #3	Average	Records
/ /						
/ /						
/ /						
/ /						
/ /						
/ /						
/ /						
/ /						
/ /						

Table 31–2   Racecar Exercise 2 Table

Date	Day #	Required Time #1	Required Time #2	Required Time #3	Average	Records
/ /						
/ /						
/ /						
/ /						
/ /						
/ /						
/ /						
/ /						
/ /						
/ /						
/ /						
/ /						
/ /						
/ /						
/ /						
/ /						
/ /						
/ /						
/ /						
/ /						
/ /						
/ /						
/ /						

Table 31–2   Racecar Exercise 2 Table (*Continued*)

Date	Day #	Required Time #1	Required Time #2	Required Time #3	Average	Records
/ /						
/ /						
/ /						
/ /						
/ /						
/ /						
/ /						
/ /						

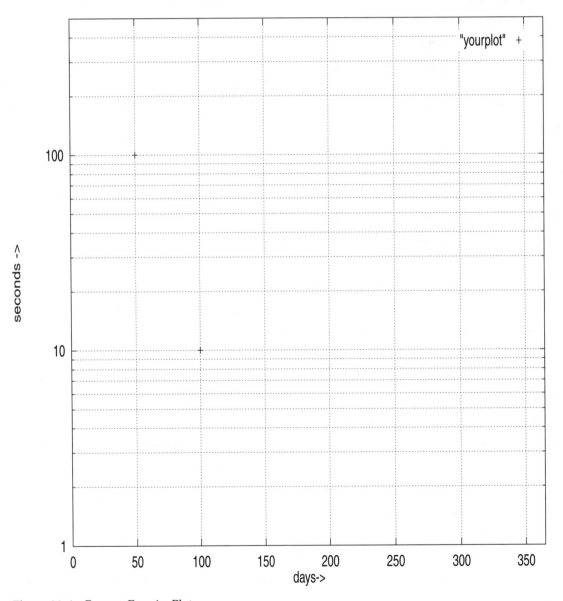

Figure 31–1   Racecar Exercise Plot

Discussion

As with the other exercises, this exercise is difficult for a stroke patient, but it really works. (And if you like car racing, you know that the drivers also have to practice many hours, just like you. If you prefer stars to cars, you know that being a star, too, requires hours of practice.)

Examples and Experiences

As you can see in Figure 31–2, the best straight line for the "Streetdress" exercise is significantly steeper than the one for "Racecar." This would imply that I was learning the "Streetdress" exercise faster than the "Racecar" exercise. This is puzzling because the exercises require the same finger movements. The only explanation I could come up with is that I always did the "Racecar" exercise first and the "Streetdress" exercise second. It could be that my affected hand considered the "Racecar" exercise as a warm up for the "Streetdress" exercise. In the figure, the upper dotted "yr" line is for the "Racecar" exercise, while the lower dotted "ys" line is for the "Streetdress" exercise. The time constant for the "Racecar" exercise was 280 days, while it was 170 days for the "Streetdress" exercise.

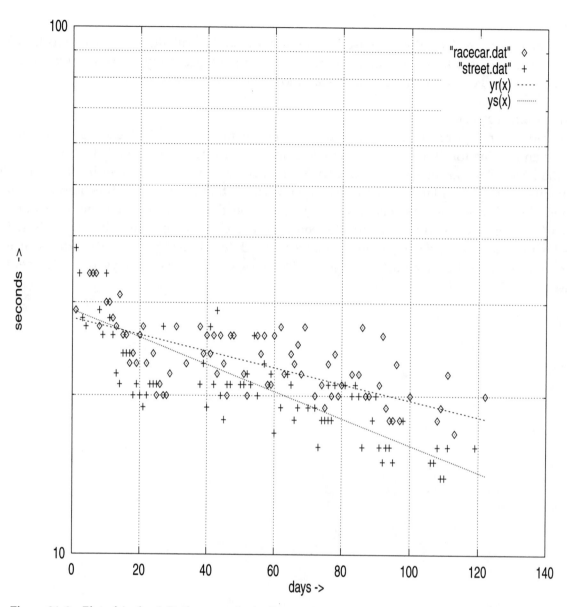

Figure 31–2 Plot of Author's Performance in the Racecar Exercise

32

Exercise 23: A Philosopher

Purpose: This exercise trains the affected hand to use all fingers individually by typing a longer sentence than in previous exercises. The sequence of the finger movements is different, more complex, and closer to random motion than in the previous exercises.

Description: In this exercise you type with both hands a poem consisting of several sentences.

When can you start to do this exercise? You can start to do this exercise when you have done "Racecar" and "Streetdress" for a week.

What do you need for this exercise? For this exercise you need a typewriter or computer keyboard. (It does not have to be functional.) If you do not have a keyboard, refer to Appendix III, "Keyboard Layout and Finger Usage," for a diagram of key placement you can use. You will also need a stopwatch that can be started, stopped, and restarted.

THE EXERCISE

1. With your unaffected hand, start the stopwatch.
2. Type the following limerick with both hands:

   A stroke-stricken philosopher in Rome
   wanted to recover at home
   so it won't be a surprise
   that he chose as exercise
   the two-handed typing of this pome.

3. When you are done, stop the stopwatch with your unaffected hand.
4. Read the stopwatch time and record it under the "Required Time #1" column in Table 32–1.
5. Repeat the entire exercise and record your time under the "Required Time #2" column in Table 32–1.
6. Repeat the entire exercise for a third time and record your time under the "Required Time #3" column in Table 32–1.

7. Calculate the average of the three required times and record it under the "Average" column in Table 32–1. If you have set a record today, congratulations! Record your score in the column labeled "Records."

8. Plot your average time in Figure 32–1. (See Chapter 9, "How to Record and Plot Your Data," for directions on plotting your data in the graph.)

9. Plot your average time in the "Overall Perspective Plot" in Chapter 36.

Table 32–1   A Philosopher Exercise Table

Date	Day #	Required Time #1	Required Time #2	Required Time #3	Average	Records
/ /						
/ /						
/ /						
/ /						
/ /						
/ /						
/ /						
/ /						
/ /						
/ /						
/ /						
/ /						
/ /						
/ /						
/ /						
/ /						
/ /						
/ /						
/ /						
/ /						
/ /						
/ /						
/ /						
/ /						
/ /						
/ /						
/ /						
/ /						
/ /						
/ /						

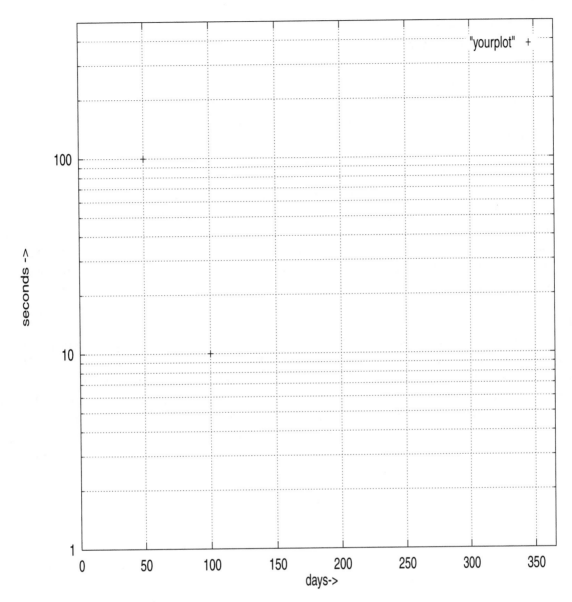

Figure 32–1   A Philosopher Exercise Plot

Discussion

British philosopher and Nobel Laureate Sir Bertrand Russell inspired this limerick. He proved that a sentence that refers to itself is meaningless. Consider the following sentence:

The woman lives in a blue house.

This sentence conveys a message. Even if I had made a typographical error; for example, if I had typed

The woman lives in a bleu house.

the contents of the sentence would still be clear. After reading the sentence you would say, "Yes, I learned something here. Not much, but something." Now compare it with the following sentence:

This sentence is grammatically correct.

After reading this sentence one realizes that it has no meaning because it refers to itself. The sentence is grammatically correct—and true—but carries no message. Russell thought up many such sentences, as did many other people. Recently, I saw this one in a student's paper:

> This sentence is wrong—oh no, on second thought, it is correct.

It is also a funny, meaningless sentence. To bring a smile to your face, I wrote a meaningless limerick for this exercise. In order for it to have meaning, you must type it a few times. Then the sentence will mean that you are recovering from a stroke!

You may notice that when you are typing this limerick, you do not bend your fingers; rather, you keep your fingers more or less stiff and move your hand so that the outstretched finger touches the keys. This is perfectly fine. Sooner or later your fingers will bend and your hand will do less of the work. For a normal person, it takes less effort to bend the fingers than to move the whole hand. For a stroke patient, however, it is the other way around. Since stroke patients have better control over the larger muscles that move their whole hand than over the smaller muscles that move their fingers, the total amount of effort is less if they move their hand rather than bend their fingers. Over time, however, the emphasis will gradually shift from moving your hand to bending your fingers.

Examples and Experiences

I originally chose a different poem to type, one written by a Dutch poet of great renown, Adriaan Roland Holst. He wrote a cycle of poems called "A Winter At Sea," which were among the best poems I have ever read. The prospect of typing a few sentences a few thousand times to train my hand led me to search for a poem that would not lose its luster after so many attempts. Of course I could type anything—a mathematical theorem, a lullaby, a prayer, an amendment to the constitution, the national anthem. Instead I chose the first verse of Holst's cycle. As it had not been translated into English, I had to translate it myself. I hope that when I have enough time I will be able to translate the whole cycle. Here is the first part:

> *Once she walked, speaking highly, along the North Sea,*
> *a day grumbled towards dawn,*
> *she shouted louder than it,*
> *still speaking with the night.*
> *Since she is fumbled by the city,*
> *on the cold of my voice,*
> *a gull climbs and moans and tumbles.*

The times I needed to type the poem can be found in Figure 32–2. The equation for the straight line is:

$$Y(t) = 85e^{-t/\tau} \tag{1}$$

where τ equals 515 days, and the point where the straight line hits the vertical axis is 85 seconds. The recovery rate time constant of 515 days indicates that after 5 times this number of days (2,575 days), I will be completely back to normal. This is roughly 8 years—a very long time, but I will get there! Notice the strange deviations on days 154 and 230. They are caused by sleeping pills I had taken the night before, which caused a remarkable slowdown the next morning in all of my exercises. Strangely enough, when I did not sleep or when I slept very poorly, there was no effect on my exercises the next morning.

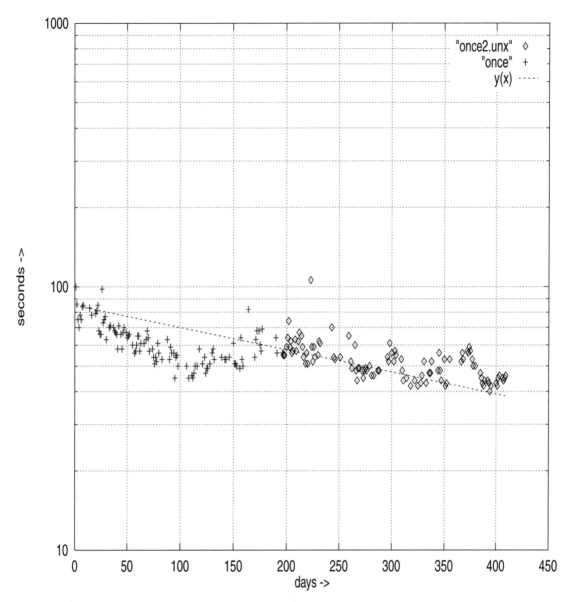

Figure 32–2 Plot of Author's Performance in the Philosopher Exercise

33

Exercise 24: A Medieval Monk

Purpose: This exercise trains the affected hand to use all fingers individually by typing a longer sentence than in previous exercises. The sequence of the finger movements is different, more complex, and closer to random motion than in the previous exercises. Also, in this exercise, no typographical errors are allowed.

Description: In this exercise you type with both hands a poem consisting of several sentences without making any typographical errors.

When can you start to do this exercise? You can start to do this exercise when you have done "Philosopher" for two weeks.

What do you need for this exercise? For this exercise you need a typewriter or computer keyboard, with a word processing software package, so you can read what you typed and count the number of typing errors.

THE EXERCISE

1. With your unaffected hand, start the stopwatch.
2. Type the following limerick with both hands, making sure that your fingers only press the keys they are supposed to press:

   A monk with a stroke in the Abbey of Montebello
   was so scared of the Abbott that he completely went psycho,
   "He will make me recopy this entire biblio,
   from beginning to end, *da capo al fino*,
   If I only make one tiny little typo."

3. When you are done, stop the stopwatch with your unaffected hand.
4. Read the stopwatch time and record it under the "Required Time #1" column in Table 33–1.
5. Count the number of errors you have made while typing. Count *all* errors, including those you made with your unaffected hand and any extra letters, spaces, or caps locks.
6. Record the number of errors under the "Errors #1" column in Table 33–2.

7. Repeat the entire exercise and record your time under the "Required Time #2" in Table 33–1 and your errors under the "Errors #2" column in Table 33–2.

8. Repeat the entire exercise and record your time under the "Required Time #3" in Table 33–1 and your errors under the "Errors #3" column in Table 33–2.

9. Calculate the average of the three required times and record it under the "Average" column in Table 33–1. If you have set a record today, congratulations! Record your score in the column labeled "Records."

10. Calculate the average of the three error measurements in the columns and record it under the "Average" column in Table 33–2. If you have set a record today, congratulations! Record your score in the column labeled "Records."

11. Plot your average time and number of errors in Figure 33–1. (See Chapter 9, "How to Record and Plot Your Data," for directions on plotting your data in the graph.)

12. Plot your average time in the "Overall Perspective Plot" in Chapter 36.

Table 33–1   A Medieval Monk Exercise Table

Date	Day #	Required Time #1	Required Time #2	Required Time #3	Average	Records
/ /						
/ /						
/ /						
/ /						
/ /						
/ /						
/ /						
/ /						
/ /						
/ /						
/ /						
/ /						
/ /						
/ /						
/ /						
/ /						
/ /						
/ /						
/ /						
/ /						
/ /						
/ /						

Table 33–1 A Medieval Monk Exercise Table (*Continued*)

Date	Day #	Required Time #1	Required Time #2	Required Time #3	Average	Records
/ /						
/ /						
/ /						
/ /						
/ /						
/ /						
/ /						
/ /						

Table 33–2 A Medieval Monk Exercise Errors Table

Date	Day #	Errors #1	Errors #2	Errors #3	Average	Records
/ /						
/ /						
/ /						
/ /						
/ /						
/ /						
/ /						
/ /						
/ /						
/ /						
/ /						
/ /						
/ /						
/ /						
/ /						
/ /						
/ /						
/ /						
/ /						
/ /						
/ /						
/ /						
/ /						

Table 33–2 A Medieval Monk Exercise Errors Table (*Continued*)

Date	Day #	Errors #1	Errors #2	Errors #3	Average	Records
/ /						
/ /						
/ /						
/ /						
/ /						
/ /						
/ /						

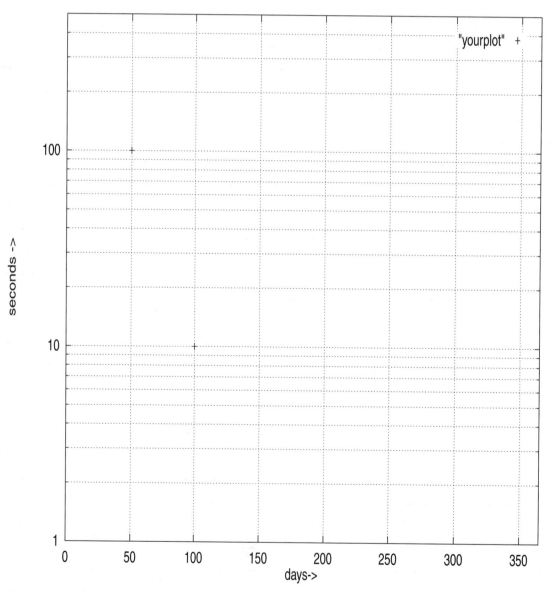

Figure 33–1 A Medieval Monk Exercise Plot (Note that this is the standard plot used for all graphs. Please ignore the fact that the y-axis reads "seconds." Consider it to read "seconds or number of errors.")

Discussion

This exercise is much more difficult than it seems. This is due to neural overflow, in which the fingers that are next to those that have to press a key also want to bend and press a key. The purpose of this exercise is to prevent this from happening.

Examples and Experiences

I had great difficulty with this exercise—more so than I expected. In other exercises in this book I ignored the quality of my performance and concentrated instead on my speed. My biggest trouble in this exercise was in bending my ring finger sufficiently. (It is needed for the W, S, and X keys.) My middle finger also gave me problems, although less than the middle finger—probably because it is stronger. The neural overflow to my ring finger was also less than it was to my middle finger. Thus, if I wanted to bend my middle finger, my ring finger bent as well, while if I wanted to bend my ring finger my middle finger bent, but not as much.

To illustrate this point, try the following experiment. Put your affected hand on the table so that it rests comfortably. Then, cock your wrist slightly, so that your fingers are all in the air, while your wrist remains on the table. Now try to move your fingers so that all fingertips touch the table. This is relatively easy. Bend your wrist up again, all fingers straight. Now try to touch the table with your middle finger while keeping all other fingers in the air. A little bending is fine, but don't let your other fingers touch the table. Difficult? Try it with all fingers keeping the others in the air. It may be impossible for you to do this. If so, don't worry; you will probably be able to do it with exercise.

As you can see in Figure 33–2, it took me about twice as much time to type without typos as it does when typos are allowed (see Exercise 23 for a comparison). Another striking feature showed up in the analysis of this exercise: While in Exercise 23 I concentrated on typing faster and was able to type faster gradually, in this exercise I concentrated on reducing the number of errors I made, or increasing the quality of my performance. Concentrating on improved quality does not automatically lead to improved speed; on the contrary, my speed remained relatively constant, although my quality improved much faster than the speed was reduced in the previous exercise. The time constant of the reduction in number of errors was 151 days, or close to one-third of the time constant of the improvement in speed of the previous exercise (which was 515 days).

There is an important lesson here: Concentration on quality leads to a small loss in speed, but also leads to a considerable increase in quality. After all, the typos you make must be corrected, which takes extra time. You may think that working towards increasing your speed and not your quality is best. I believe it is the other way around: working on improving quality is more important than is improving speed. You can improve your quality by concentrating, slowing down a bit, and paying extra attention to what you do. These mental efforts do little to increase speed, but they do increase the quality with little harm to speed. Thus, *it is better to emphasize quality than speed.*

Notice that the time it took me to finish this exercise (the upper series of points) does not change much. However, the number of errors (the lower series of points) goes down steadily. The time constant for the reduction in number of errors was 151 days. This is much smaller than the time constant of 515 days for the reduction in required time in the previous exercise.

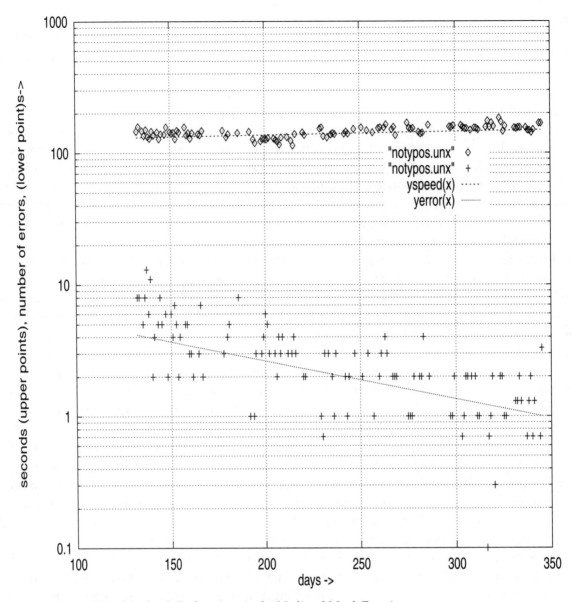

Figure 33–2   Plot of Author's Performance in the Medieval Monk Exercise

34

Exercise 25: Thumb to Joints

Purpose: This exercise develops motion of the tip of the thumb.

Description: In this exercise you touch the joints of your index finger with your thumb. In doing so, you make forward and sideways motions.

When can you start to do this exercise? You can start to do this exercise immediately after your outpatient rehabilitation therapy has ended.

What do you need for this exercise? For this exercise you need a stopwatch that can be started, stopped, and restarted.

THE EXERCISE

1. Start the stopwatch and put your affected hand with its back in the palm of your unaffected hand.
2. Move the index finger of your affected hand so that its backside rests against the inside of the index finger of your unaffected hand.
3. Move the thumb of your unaffected hand such that it rests against the inside of the index finger of your affected hand. Now the index finger of your affected hand can be firmly held between the thumb and index finger of your unaffected hand. You can hold it still by squeezing it. Make sure that the side of the index finger of your affected hand is still visible and can be easily touched. The thumb of your affected hand is sticking in the air.
4. Move the tip of the thumb of your affected hand to the tip of the index finger of your affected hand. I know that this sounds easy, but it is probably impossible for you, like it was impossible for me when I started to do this exercise. If you cannot do it, you may help the affected hand with your unaffected hand by pushing the tip of the thumb of your affected hand with the thumb of your unaffected hand against the tip of the index finger of your affected hand. (I hope that you can still follow me after this convoluted explanation!) You may move your wrist on the affected side; you may bend the index finger of the affected side; but don't let it slip out of the grip of the index finger and thumb of your unaffected hand.

5. Pull the thumb of your affected hand back so that it sticks in the air again. Pull it back as far as you can, so that the opening between your thumb and index finger is as wide as possible. This also sounds very easy but is equally difficult. Once your brain has figured out what you want to do with your thumb, it will begin to move it very gradually.

6. Now move the tip of your thumb to the first joint of the index finger (counted down from the tip). This is the joint that connects the last bone of your finger to the center bone of the finger. (These bones are each called the *phalanx.*)

7. Again, pull the thumb of your affected hand back so that it sticks in the air. Pull it back as far as you can so that the opening between your thumb and index finger is as wide as possible.

8. Move the tip of your thumb to the second joint of the index finger (counting from the tip down).

9. Pull the thumb back as far as possible one more time. You have now touched the thumb to the index finger 3 times.

10. Now, touch these spots on the index finger 20 times each (that is, make 60 touches, or 20 sets of 3 touches). Count from 1 to 60 while doing so. You may walk around while doing this, just be back in time to stop the stopwatch.

11. Stop the stopwatch and record the time under the "Required Time" column in Table 34–1. If you have set a record today, congratulations! Record your score in the column labeled "Records."

12. Plot your time in Figure 34–1. (See Chapter 9, "How to Record and Plot Your Data," for directions on plotting your data in the graph.)

13. Plot your average time in the "Overall Perspective Plot" in Chapter 36.

Table 34–1   Thumb to Joints Exercise Table

Date	Day #	Required Time	Records
/ /			
/ /			
/ /			
/ /			
/ /			
/ /			
/ /			
/ /			
/ /			
/ /			
/ /			
/ /			
/ /			
/ /			
/ /			
/ /			

Table 34–1   Thumb to Joints Exercise Table (*Continued*)

Date	Day #	Required Time	Records
/ /			
/ /			
/ /			
/ /			
/ /			
/ /			
/ /			
/ /			
/ /			
/ /			
/ /			
/ /			
/ /			
/ /			
/ /			

Discussion

This exercise is so hard that you may be unable to complete it. In particular, you may find that pulling your thumb back is difficult. You may be able to do it 10 or 20 times, but not 60 times. This is normal, so don't be discouraged. If you cannot complete the exercise with the thumb working by itself, then help your thumb with your unaffected hand. There are two parts to each movement: the thumb moving forward and pulling back. The first motion is accomplished by the muscles in the thenar eminens (the bulbous part of the hand near the base of the thumb). These are relatively short, thick muscles in normal people, but they may have shrunk or flattened in your hand because of your stroke. The second motion is performed by two muscles located on the upper side of the forearm. Since muscles closest to the brain recover fastest, these muscles have recovered a bit more than those in the thenar eminens.

It may feel like the muscles in your thenar eminens are made of barbed wire, and that these barbed wires are moving inside tender tissue, making this exercise very painful. If the pain gets too bad, stop doing the exercise. However, don't give up on this exercise completely; you need your thumb later in life. This exercise may also take a long time to finish. That is why it is done only once per session. You may notice after a while that your thumb bends at its first joint. Normal people can bend their thumb at the first and second joint (counting from the tip down). Try bending your thumb at the second joint only, keeping the first joint straight. This motion is required in such elementary tasks as picking up a plate or a cup and saucer.

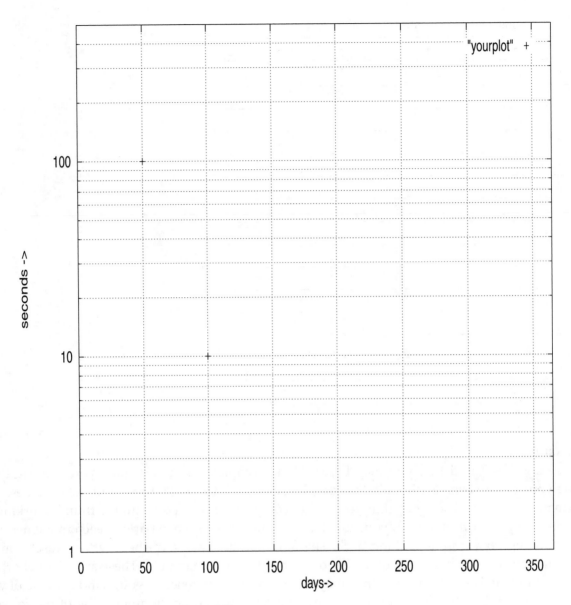

Figure 34–1 Thumb to Joints Exercise Plot

35

Exercise 26: Twenty-Nine Facial Exercises

Purpose: This exercise stimulates your facial muscles to promote the formation of facial expressions.
Description: In this exercise you move muscles of the face to move parts of the face.
When can you start to do this exercise? You can start to do this exercise as soon as you feel like it, as no particular skills are used.
What do you need for this exercise? For this exercise you need a mirror, a pencil, and a stopwatch that can be started, stopped, and restarted.

THE EXERCISE

First read the exercises carefully and try them a few times. If you are unable to perform a certain exercise because of paralysis, don't worry about it. Spend as much time *thinking* your way through the exercise as you would if you were actually *doing* it. Gradually, your brain will figure out what you want and will do it. You have to give it time though. Keep a pencil around so that you can keep track of which exercise you are on; there are quite a few, and you may get confused over which exercise is next. Each exercise should be repeated 20 times.

Note: The point where the middle of your upper lip touches the middle of your lower lip is called the mid-lip point.

1. Sit in front of a mirror.
2. Start the stopwatch with your unaffected hand.
3. Move your mid-lip point forward, away from your teeth, as if you are sucking on a straw or as if you are going to kiss someone.
4. Move your mid-lip point as close as you can towards your teeth.
5. Move your mid-lip point as far as you can to the left.
6. Move your mid-lip point as far as you can to the right.
7. Move your mid-lip point as far as you can to your affected side, and let it go back to its central position. In one long, flowing movement, take the mid-lip point to the farthest point on the unaffected side.

8. Move your mid-lip point as far as you can to the affected side and hold it there. While it is there, move the mid-lip point forwards, like you are trying to kiss someone who is not in front of you, but a little bit on the side.

9. Move your mid-lip point all the way to the other side and again hold it there and move it forward as far as you can.

10. Move your mid-lip point as far as you can to the left and hold it. Move it forward as if you are kissing someone to your left, then in one long, flowing movement move your mid-lip point to the right, and move it forward again, as if you are kissing a second person who is touching cheeks with the first person.

11. Pull both corners of your mouth down as far as you can, making the grimmest possible face.

12. Pull both corners of your mouth up as high as you can, making the happiest possible face.

13. Pull both corners of your mouth as far as you can to your ears, making the widest possible smile.

14. Imagine pushing the skin of your face up with your hand, as if you are stroking your own face upward. Now try to accomplish the same motion of the skin, but without touching it with your hand. Use your facial muscles only.

15. Move the tip of your nose down as far as you can.

16. Move the tip of your nose to the left. You may not be able to do this because of your paralysis, but give it a try.

17. Move the tip of your nose to the right.

18. Open your eyes as wide as you can.

19. Raise your eyebrows as high as you can.

A stroke patient in Plaistow
who did not have a lot of know-how,
went after his recovery
straight to a university
Saying: "I am now a trained high-brow"

20. Raise your right eyebrow only.

21. Raise your left eyebrow only.

22. Pull your ears backward. (If you cannot do this, just skip this part.)

A stroker in the town of Triers,
was faced with suspicion by his peers,
"You always swim faster,
how do you do that, you little lame baster' "
He said: "I have learned how to swim with my ears"

23. Pull your ears upward. (Again, you may not be able to do this; if not, skip this part.) You may notice that if you pull your ears upwards, your eyebrows move upwards too, as if you are pulling the center of your scalp upwards, and everything follows that upward motion.

24. Stick your tongue out as far as you can. Move it from left to right as far as you can, like a windshield wiper on a car on a rainy day.

25. Stick your tongue out as far as you can and try to touch the tip of your nose, then try to touch the tip of your chin.

26. Close both eyes, then open only the left one.

27. Close both eyes, then open only the right one.
28. With both eyes open, close only your left one. Try to keep your right eye open.
29. With both eyes open, close only your right one. Try to keep your left eye open.
30. When you have done all of the above exercises 20 times, you can stop the stopwatch.
31. Record the time it took you to finish this exercise in Table 35–1.
32. Plot your time in Figure 35–1. (See Chapter 9, "How to Record and Plot Your Data," for directions on plotting your data in the graph.)
33. Plot your average time in the "Overall Perspective Plot" in Chapter 36.

Table 35–1 *Twenty-Nine Facial Exercises Table*

Date	Day #	Required Time	Records
/ /			
/ /			
/ /			
/ /			
/ /			
/ /			
/ /			
/ /			
/ /			
/ /			
/ /			
/ /			
/ /			
/ /			
/ /			
/ /			
/ /			
/ /			

Discussion

When you do these exercises, you should expect to experience many associate movements. This is because the volume of the part of the brain that is charged with control over the face is so large. If this exercise makes you uncomfortable, ignore it completely.

Examples and Experiences

In reviewing textbooks on the subject of recovery, I have found no consensus on what to do with the associate movements caused by this exercise. Some researchers recommend that they be suppressed because they cause extra muscle tension. Others recommend exploiting them to help in the rehabilitation process. Whatever their application, the verdict is still out on how to use them or how effective they are.

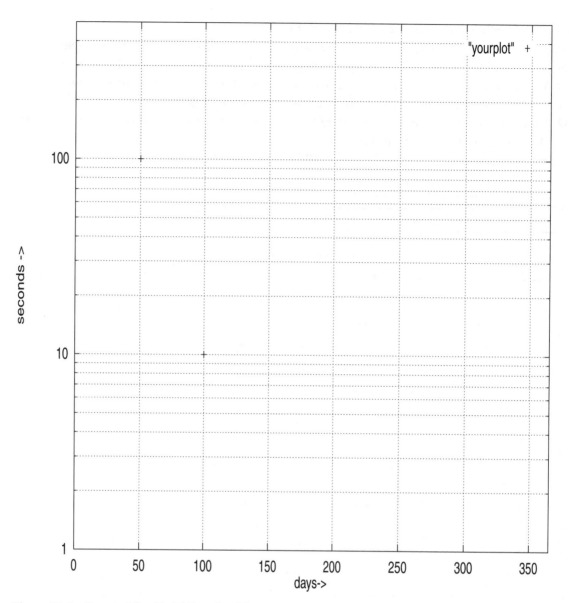

Figure 35–1   Twenty-Nine Facial Exercises Plot

During the face push-up, I noticed that my affected side index finger became strongly bent (due to neural overflow). I actually had to straighten it forcefully with my unaffected hand in order to continue. This bending would be so strong that my tendons were quite painful. I found the exercise in which both eyes are closed and then the right eye is opened impossible to do. I could not keep my left eye closed when I opened my right eye. Instead, my small toe curled strongly inward, so that my foot rested on the ground on my small toe only. The exercise in which you open the left eye while keeping the right eye closed was a piece of cake for me, but the other way around was impossible. The exercise in which both eyes are open and you have to close your left eye produces a very strange result: my left arm (the affected arm) started to turn with the palm up. Another strange effect occurred during the entire face push-up. I felt a sharp pain next to my thumbnail on my affected side.

In all of these facial exercises I felt one or more associate movements—often very subtle, sometimes very strong—with one exception: the tongue sweep exercise. In this exercise, nothing unusual happened (which may be unusual in its own right).

36

The Overall Perspective

In this chapter you will combine all the plots you have made into one plot. Looking at all of your work displayed in one plot will give you a sense of satisfaction and achievement, while it will also give you some assurance that your recovery is going well. On the other hand, if all is not going well (for example, if you have had a hidden stroke), it will probably show up in this plot as well. If you have changed your daily routine, this may also show up in the plot. It is important to note that a small change, such as doing the exercises in a different order, may have considerable consequences.

I described in Chapter 7 that it worked best for me to do the two ball-catching exercises last on any given day. The reason was that in these exercises, the ball hits the hand some 200 times, sending a torrent of sensory impulses at every hit to the area of the brain that has been wiped out by the stroke. Neighboring areas of the brain must help out. These areas of the brain are trying to figure out what to do to help you catch the balls. This is a pretty big task for them. When the 200 sensory pulses further confuse these areas, they may become overloaded and not function well if you try to do the pencil exercises next. If I did the pencil exercises before the ball exercises, the former went much better than if the order was reversed. You may have a different area of the brain that is affected, and this example may not be valid for you. Try to figure out what the best order is for you. In the overall perspective you will quickly notice when something is amiss, and you can immediately change your routine.

The overall perspective plot may help you decide whether to take a break from the exercises for a couple of days or a week. When you resume your exercises after the break, you may notice that you have deteriorated. This deterioration may be different in different exercises; it may not be all that serious; or it may be quite dramatic. I once took an out-of-state trip that resulted in my suspending my exercises for 10 days. When I resumed exercising I found that I had deteriorated 20 to 50 percent, depending on the exercise. It took me more than two weeks to reverse the deterioration to my performances on the day when the suspension began.

Also, as I mentioned in Chapter 4, when I changed my endurance exercise from 10 minutes on an exercise bike to a one-hour walk, I experienced a profoundly negative effect on my performances. You may encounter a similar situation. Without an overall perspective plot, you may not notice this setback, and may in turn suffer an unnecessary delay in your recovery process. I lost at least three months in my recovery process by not knowing the superiority of the exercise bike as an endurance exercise. I found this out by comparing all my exercise plots.

What and How to Plot on Your Overall Perspective Plot

Since your overall perspective plot will become very crowded, it helps if the information is as clean as possible. I found that it works best to use different colors for different exercises. I suggest you use a set of multicolored felt-tip pens or colored pencils. You should also buy a small container of white-out to cover mistakes.

To mark a point in the plot, use a single small dot—don't use plus signs, crosses, or small circles, as they will overlap. I suggest you use the color scheme found in Table 36–1, or feel free to create a color scheme of your own. Once you choose your scheme, write it down and stick to it; otherwise you will get very confused. You may then plot your results in Figure 36–1 (for your first year) or Figure 36–2 (for your second year).

Table 36–1   Color Scheme for the Overall Perspective Plot

Catch a Bouncer	Red
Ball from Left to Right	Blue
Ball Back in Hand	Green
Ten Pencils, Mug-to-Mug	Black
Ten Pencils, Mug-to-Table-to-Mug	Red
Turn a Pencil Clockwise	Blue
Turn a Pencil Counterclockwise	Green
Ten Pencils, Eraser-End First	Black
QW	Red
QWT	Blue
THREE	Green
FOUR	Black
FIVE	Red
WAFERS10/MONOPOLY10	Green
The Quick Fox	Black
Racecar	Red
Streetdress	Blue
A Philosopher	Green
A Medieval Monk (time)	Black
A Medieval Monk (number of errors)	Red
Twenty-Nine Facial Exercises	Black

Examples and Experiences

In Figure 36–3, you can see my recovery process for two years. After two years I had gone through two time constants in all of my exercises, and I had recovered around 80 percent of my normal capacity. I then decided to quit all exercises except three: the bike exercise and the ball-catching exercises. These provide a great deal of movement and activation for my arm and hand. Further recovery came from my daily activities.

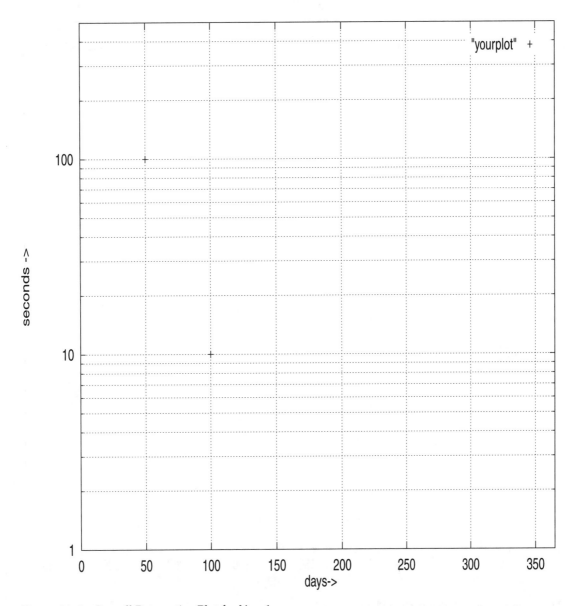

Figure 36–1   Overall Perspective Plot for Year 1

Since I did not have a workbook to start with, I did not make an overall plot until later in the program. I had also wrongly chosen the first day of each exercise as day 1 for that exercise, so my exercises were out of synch. Nevertheless, I found that the best solution was to combine all the graphs I made in Figure 36–3. Notice that I show improvement in all exercises, but that I also suffered from the change I made in my endurance exercise.

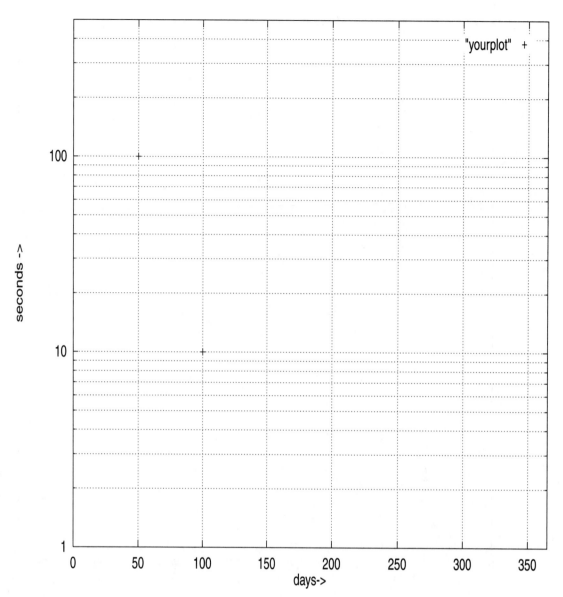

Figure 36–2   Overall Perspective Plot for Year 2

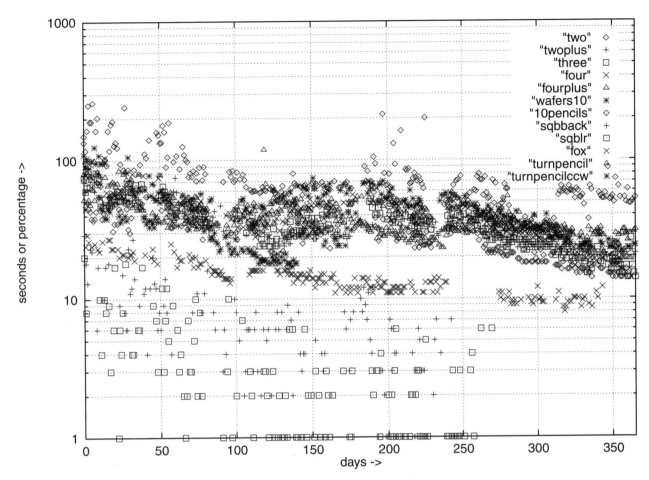

Figure 36–3   Overall Perspective of the Author's Recovery Process for One Year

37

When to Make the Transition to a Maintenance Program

After you have performed your exercises for a couple of months you may wonder when you can quit doing them. I, too, wondered about this and came to the conclusion that after I had performed any particular exercise for a length of time equal to one time constant, I had regained about 63 percent of my normal capacities. After two time constants, I had reached 87 percent. That is not 100 percent or even 99 percent. However, the hand will continue to recover if it is used for daily living activities. Thus, I terminated an exercise after two time constants. As all exercises have different time constants, the time at which an exercise can be stopped varies. You can learn more about determining time constants in Appendix IV.

To make sure that my hand stays fit, I perform a daily maintenance program. This maintenance program consists of a number of exercises described in this book:

1. Exercise 0, The Bike
2. Exercise 7, Ball from Left to Right
3. Exercise 8, Ball Back in Hand

Appendix I

About the Authors

Johannes (Jan) Smits and Else (Els) Smits-Boone are husband and wife, both born and raised in the Netherlands. Els was educated at the Academy of Fine Arts in Amsterdam in ceramics, drawing, and painting. She has had over twenty one-person and group exhibitions of her work, in Europe and North America. Her work has been acquired by private collectors and art museums. Her favorite medium is pen-and-ink drawings, with finely drawn lines of textured imaginary spaces and objects, and dream-like figures and animals, especially cats. The fact that she has four cats accounts for the fact that many of her drawings are of frolicking cats. She is also an excellent cook, and has written a cookbook (*The Artist's Cookbook*) with an eclectic mixture of Dutch and American recipes.

Els dropped these activities when Jan had his stroke in order to help him with his recovery. She was the creative person who invented the majority of the exercises in this book. She persuaded Jan, often against his will, to try some of the exercises. He was often convinced that the exercises would be too difficult, and would thus reject an idea for an exercise out of hand. Although this was his initial reaction, he did try the exercises eventually. Some were indeed too difficult, so their performance was postponed until a time when he was able to do them.

Jan received his Doctorandus degree in Physics at the University of Leyden, and his Ph.D. in Electrical Engineering from the University of Twente. He joined the faculty at Boston University in 1985, and has worked there since then in the College of Engineering in the Department of Electrical and Computer Engineering. Here he specializes in microelectro-mechanical devices. He worked on silicon processing for micromachines, and on thin film piezoelectric materials. He fabricated micro-pumps for drug delivery systems and made the first commercially available micromachined optical scanners. He is also a Fellow of the Institute of Electrical and Electronic Engineers.

In the summer of 1995, Jan suffered a severe stroke due to a dissection of the carotid artery. His ability to measure the properties of microscopically small devices prepared him well for the measurements of the minute changes as they occur in the performances of a stroke patient. So while Els came up with the ideas on which exercises to perform, he came up with the ideas on what to measure, how to record it, and how to analyze the results. In the course of his work, he had often seen naturally occurring exponential decay functions, and he was not surprised that the underlying function in the recovery process was another manifestation of this natural process.

Appendix II

The Scientific Report about the Method as Described in this Book

Here follows the complete text of the scientific report as it was published in the *Journal of Neurovascular Disease* (September–October 1997, pages 211–219). This paper is presented with permission of the publisher of the *Journal of Neurovascular Disease*, Prime National Publishing Corporation, of Weston, Massachusetts. Some of the names of the exercises have been changed in this book from how they appeared in the paper, but the change in name does not refer to a change in the exercises themselves.

Recovery Rate Constants of Recovery from Stroke

J.G. Smits, Ph.D.

ABSTRACT
BACKGROUND AND PURPOSE

A stroke patient performed a set of 18 exercises during 24 months, recording and making plots of his performance. His exercises were aimed at improvement in four areas: manipulation of medium-size objects, improvement of eye-hand coordination, movement and control of individual fingers, movement and control of the thumb. The patient devised the exercises, executed them, and measured his own performance. Therefore this paper is the result of self-observation of the patient.

METHODS

In some exercises it was determined how long it took to perform each task with a stopwatch, while in other exercises the quality of the performance, determined as the number of errors occurring during the execution of a task, was measured.

RESULTS

The performances could be described as exponential decay functions, regardless of whether the performance was measured as the time required to execute a certain task or as the error percentage in a task in which quality of performance was measured. Each task had its own time constant, the recovery rate time constant for that task. The recovery rate time constants have been measured for all tasks; they ranged from 85 days to 267 days. The tasks were arranged according to complexity, determined by the number of subtasks in each of the tasks. The measured time constants were plotted versus the complexity and a linear regression was performed. It was found that the time constants were approximately linearly proportional to the complexity. Every subtask added about 29 days to the time constants.

CONCLUSIONS

No leveling-off to a plateau was observed, instead, every performance was approximately a straight line in a log-line plot. The recovery process was rather predictable.

Keywords: Exercises, Rehabilitation, Outcome, Recovery-Rate.

INTRODUCTION

It is widely believed that stroke patients who survive stroke, but who are hemiplegic, can be rehabilitated somewhat, with most of the rehabilitation occurring in the first three to six months after the stroke. Health insurance companies take this into consideration when a patient requests more rehabilitation. Sometimes, requests for continued rehabilitation are turned down by the insurer when a patient has had a few months of OT or PT based on the belief that more therapy will not be helpful.

In this report, a scientist who suffered a stroke and received PT and OT for three months, but who felt that he needed more rehabilitation (which was denied by his insurance company), reports about his self-designed exercises, by which he was able to continue his recovery and also to prove that his recovery continued exponentially with the amount of time spent in exercising.

He designed a large number of exercises, which satisfied the following criteria:

- they had to be easily reproducible,
- they had to be easily and accurately measurable,
- they had to be relevant to recovery, and
- they could not overly fatigue the patient or induce spasticity.

As physicist and engineer, the author decided to tackle the problem of his recovery in the same way as he would approach any other scientific problem: by studying the literature, designing experiments to measure certain variables, analyze the results, draw conclusions, and implement changes to get improvements. While in the process of recording and analyzing his performance it became clear that his performances as measured in his exercises were exponential decay functions. These are functions that contain a time dependent factor $e^{-t/\tau}$, in which t is the time and τ is called the time constant of the process. They derive their name from the decay in radiation levels of radioactive materials, which contains the same time dependent factor. If the radiation level of these materials is measured at a time t_0, and the radiation level is called 100 percent of a reference level R_0, then after a lapse of time t equal to the time constant τ, the exponential has reached the value $e^{-\tau/\tau} = e^{-1} = 0.37$, so the radiation level is then at 37 percent of R_0. When the radiation levels are measured as function of time, and plotted in a semi-logarithmic plot, they show a straight line, of which the slope is equal to $1/\tau$. As the same feature shows up in the present measurements, it can be concluded that the same temporal dependence plays a role, since this is the only function that shows this behavior. Other examples of these exponential decay functions are the water level in a leaking bucket, the pressure in a leaking tire, or the voltage on a capacitor that is discharged through a resistor. In all cases, the time constant τ can be expressed in the parameters of the system; in the case of the leaking bucket, the time constant is equal to the product of the capacity of the bucket and the water resistance of the leak. Larger buckets and larger resistance both lead to longer time constants. The fact that the same time dependence shows up in this case indicates that a similar process may be going on, where the capacity of the bucket is the analogon of the total amount of neurons associated with the performance of the task, and the resistance is a measure of the difficulty of the task. The time constants of all exercises have been determined and compared, the relative difficulty, here called complexity, of the tasks has been determined as the number of subtasks in any given task, and the speculation implied in the previous statement has been tested and found to be plausible.

An interesting aspect of these measurements is that the time constant could be determined after a few weeks, and that the recovery continued for hundreds of days as predicted by the initial determination of the time constant. This made the recovery process extremely predictable.

The first purpose of the present investigation was to find whether the leveling-off as is reported to occur after three to six months is due to the fact that exercises are no longer performed or if there is a natural barrier that cannot be overcome, regardless of the effort. The second purpose of this investigation was to gather a large amount of measurements, which would enable us to study the experimental data statistically by using mathematical models. Surprisingly, the exponential decay character of the performances although unanticipated, showed up very clearly. An observation was that the time constants of the decay curves depend approximately linearly on the complexity of the exercise.

THE SUBJECT

Although this report has been written in the third person, it is the result of self observation by the author, who is both observer and subject.

The subject was a 51-year-old white male, 1.72 meters tall, weighing 62 kg. He was a physicist with a Ph.D. in Electrical Engineering. He suffered a stroke due to a dissection of the right internal carotid, which could have been induced by a sudden head motion while falling asleep on a transatlantic night flight. He was admitted to a hospital where he was administered heparin, and later coumadin. He had no sensation on his left side and no motor control over any muscle on the left side of his body. Earlier that day he had complained about a severe headache for which he had taken aspirin, and he had noticed dim vision and the appearance of bright floating objects in his field of view. He had also complained about loss of peripheral vision on the underside of his field of view. He regained some motion in his shoulder and arm in four days and in his affected leg in seven days.

In the first three weeks after the stroke he was unable to read as he could not coordinate the motion of both eyes. He did not remember the entire alphabet, just bits and pieces. By way of checking up on himself, he tried to derive the differential equation of a vibrating beam and solve it in the hospital—a subject he had been working on shortly before the stroke. He did appear to have considerable cognitive deficits. He also had a severe left neglect, not noticing objects on his left side (e.g., forgetting to shave the left side of the face, leaving the shaving lather untouched, even though he looked in a mirror). He did recognize his near relatives and friends, but not the faces of famous people and celebrities (presidents, news anchors, movie stars).

After one week in intensive care he was moved to a rehabilitation hospital where he underwent occupational and physical therapy for three weeks as an in-patient, and subsequently for three months as an outpatient. When his treatment ended, he was able to walk without help and climb stairs with help, he was able to close his affected fist but was not able to open it. His strength was enough to support an empty briefcase. His dexterity was insufficient to pick up a pencil, a ball, a drinking glass, or other medium-sized objects, or to flip a light switch, hold a knife or fork or pencil, or to tie his shoelaces. He experienced extreme sensitivity to noise (hyperacusie) as alluded to in [11].

THE EXERCISES

He performed the following exercises every day:

- **Endurance**

  1. He exercised on an exercise bike with hand and foot pedals for 10 minutes, (day 1 through day 120 and day 260 through day 365).
  2. He walked in the neighborhood for 1 hour (day 120 through day 260).

- **Eye-Hand Coordination and Hand Exercise**

  1. (BALL LR) Throwing a ball up with the unaffected (right) hand and catching it with the affected (left) hand. This was repeated 100 times and the number of missed catches was recorded.
  2. (Ball Back in Hand) Throwing a ball up with the affected hand and catching it with the affected hand, again repeated 100 times with the number of missed catches recorded.

- **Manipulation of Medium-Sized Objects**

  1. (10 Pencils Mug-to-Mug) He put 10 pencils in a coffee mug, took them out one by one and put them in an empty mug all with his affected hand. The time to complete the exercise was recorded.
  2. (10 Pencils Mug-to-Table-to-Mug) He put 10 pencils in a mug, took them out one by one, dropped them on the table, picked them up, and put them back in the mug, tip forward. The time to complete the exercise was recorded.
  3. (10 Pencils, Eraser-End First) Same as the above exercise, but now putting the pencil in the mug with the backside first. He had to extend the wrist, while holding on to the pencil, letting it go with the wrist extended.

4. (Turnpencil) He put a pencil on the table with the tip pointing away from him, he picked it up and put it down with the tip towards him, turning the pencil clockwise. Repeated 20 times and recorded the time required.

5. (Turn a Pencil Counterclockwise) Same as above but rotating the pencil counterclockwise.

• Exercises to Move Fingers Individually

1. (TWO) On a computer keyboard, he pressed all sets of two neighboring letter keys with index finger and middle finger. Recorded the time to press all pairs. [In the book this is referred to as QW.]

2. (TWOPLUS) Same as above but followed by a touch on the spacebar with the thumb of the affected hand. [In the book this is referred to as QWT.]

3. (THREE) On a computer keyboard, he touched all sets of three neighboring keys, with index finger, middle finger, and ring finger. Recorded the time to press all sets of three neighboring keys.

4. (FOUR) Similarly pressed all sets of four neighboring keys with index finger, middle finger, ring finger, and little finger. Recorded time for all sets of four neighbors.

5. (FOURPLUS) Like the previous exercise, but now followed by touching the spacebar with the thumb. [In the book this is referred to as FIVE.]

6. (MRL) He pressed all letter keys on a computer keyboard with the middle finger, ring finger, or little finger only. Recorded the required times. [This exercise was not included in the book as it was found to not be a good exercise.]

7. (WAFERS10) He typed a word for which only the left hand was required. [Since his work involved silicon wafers, he chose "wafers."] He typed it 10 times, every time followed by the numeral indicating how many times he had typed it, to avoid making errors due to skipping it. Measured the required time.

8. (Racecar, Streetdress) He typed two sentences with the left hand exclusively, using only the left side of the keyboard. These were: "We were raw, scarred racers, we raced sacred racecars fastest" and "We ex-stars wear streetdresses at crazy catered fests." Recorded the required time.

• For Integration of Left and Right Hand

1. (Fox) He typed the sentence "The quick brown fox jumps over the lazy dog" since it contains all letter of the alphabet. Recorded the required time.

2. (Once She Walked) He typed with both hands a six-line poem by the poet Adriaan Roland Holst. Recorded the required time. [In the book this is referred to as "A Philosopher."]

• Exercises for the Thumb

1. (Thumb to Joints) He brought the tip of the thumb to the tip and the two joints of the index finger, repeated it 20 times, recorded time it required.

2. (Thumbphone) On a hand-held phone, with the keys on the inside of the handset he held the phone in the affected hand and pressed all numbers three times with the thumb, recorded required time. [This exercise is not in the book as it was found not to be a good exercise.]

DISCUSSION

It was observed that the times required for the exercises gradually decreased. Since there was considerable scatter in the data, the nature of the function to describe the recovery was not immediately clear, but it became obvious that they must be exponential decay functions when the data were plotted on a log scale. Exponential decay functions contain $e^{-t/\tau}$ as in

$$P(t) = P_n + (P_0 - P_n)e^{-t}/\tau \qquad (1)$$

in which $P(t)$ is the performance as function of the time t, where $P(t)$ is measured as the required time for the exercises or as the percentage of balls missed in the catching exercises; t is the time since the beginning of the exercises, it is measured as the number of days since the first performance of the exercise; P_0 is the performance at the first day; and P_n is the performance of a normal person. The time constant τ is the characteristic element in this equation. After a period of time equal to one time constant, the exponential drops to $e^{-1} = 0.37$, while after 4.5 time constants it drops to around 0.01. The function $P(t)$ approaches P_n asymptotically. For practical purposes, it is satisfactory to assume that after five time constants (when its actual value is 0.0067) the exponential decay function is equal to zero. In the case that

$$P_0 \gg P_n \text{ and } t \ll \tau \qquad (2)$$

equation (1) may be approximated by

$$P(t) = P_0 e_{-t\backslash\tau} \qquad (3)$$

Even though P_n is not known for the exercises, it is clear that the inequality in expression (2) holds, which enables us to determine τ.

Most exercises showed an initial period with much scatter, and very little, if any, improvement. It was theorized that this initial period is a random trial and error period in which the subject tries to find out how to perform the exercise. The scatter gradually diminished, and in all exercises a period of consistent improvement began. A similar effect has been observed in squirrel monkeys who had received a brain lesion by electro-coagulation [10].

One exercise (10 Pencils, Mug-to-Table-to-Mug) showed an initial improvement, like all other exercises, but also a dramatic deterioration, which did not occur in the other exercises. In this exercise the subject picks up a pencil to put it in a mug. After roughly 200 days, he dropped the pencil more and more frequently, making it difficult to finish the exercise. It was observed that the picking of the pencil occurred with the index finger and thumb, while the middle finger, due to bending from neural overflow, pushed the pencil out of reach. A similar deterioration has been observed in the previously mentioned squirrel monkeys that pick up food pellets from small wells [10].

On the log scale plots, the performance can be approximated by a straight line, of which the slope is $-1/\tau$. This enabled us to measure the time constant τ for each of the exercises. To do this a linear regression on the measurement data was performed after the logarithms were taken.

In Figure APII–1 the performance for exercises TWO, TWOPLUS, THREE, FOUR and FOUR-PLUS have been plotted for the first 120 days, together with the linear best fit [y2(x), y2p(x), y3(x), y4(x), y4p(x)] in the log scale plots.

The results for the time constant calculations showed that every exercise had its own time constant. The smallest time constant was 85 days (for BALL LR), the largest was 267 days (for WAFERS10). Since the functions drop to 0.6 percent in five time constants, it is presumed that after $5\backslash\tau$ the patient has recovered completely, so we call $t_{etr} = 5\tau$ the Expected Total Recovery Time. This

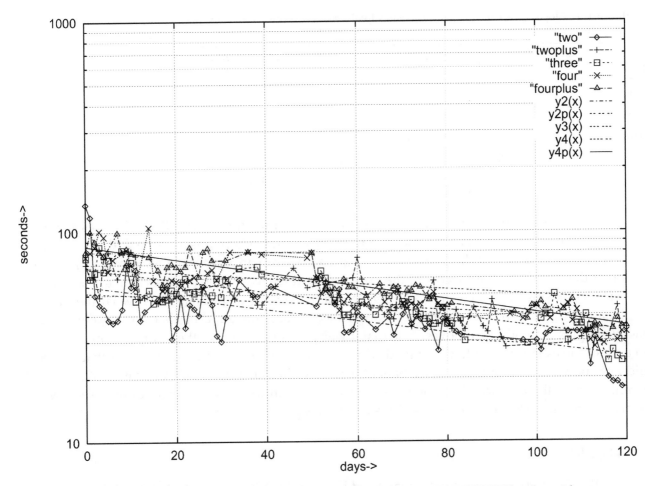

Figure ApII–1   Performance in Exercises TWO, TWOPLUS, THREE, FOUR, and FOURPLUS Together with the Best Fits y2(x), y2p(x), y3(x), y4(x), and y4p(x)

leads to t_{etr} values in the range of 425 days and 1,335 days respectively (BALL LR and WAFERS10). It should be noted that a stroke patient has to maintain his exercise regime during this time period, otherwise the recovery rate time constant and the expected recovery time may change.

In Table ApII–1, for each exercise the slopes, time constants, and expected total recovery times (as measured after 365 days of exercising) is provided.

Table ApII–1   Slope, Time Constant, and Expected Total Recovery Time for Each Exercise

Exercise	Slope	Time Constant τ[Days]	Expected Total Recovery Time (5τ) [Days]
10pencils	-0.00754	132	663
Turnpencil	-0.00689	145	726
TWO	-0.00506	197	998
TWOPLUS	-0.00547	182	914
THREE	-0.0054	185	925
FOUR	-0.00494	202	1,010

Table ApII–1   Slope, Time Constant, and Expected Total Recovery Time for Each Exercise (*Continued*)

Exercise	Slope	Time Constant τ[Days]	Expected Total Recovery Time (5τ) [Days]
FOURPLUS	-0.00524	190	950
WAFERS10	-0.00374	267	1,335
ballLR	-0.0118	85	425
ballback	-0.00926	107	535
fox	-0.0032	309	1,545

It should be noted that at the total expected recovery time for exercise BALL LR was 425 days. This paper has been finished at day 430, and the subject can perform this exercise with normal quality (zero missed catches) at this moment (his first-day performance was 80 missed catches), an indication of the validity of the concept of the expected total recovery time for a particular exercise.

The large spread in recovery rate time constants spurred a speculation on what the possible explanation could be of this divergence. A possible explanation could be that some exercises were more complex than others. To investigate that it was pondered whether the number of muscles used in each of the exercises should be counted. This idea was discarded when we realized that we really did not know which muscles a stroke patient uses since he can accomplish a certain task using different muscles than a normal person does. Instead, to quantify the complexity of the exercises, we analyzed the subtasks in each exercise. This analysis is presented here.

SUBTASKS

- (Ball LR) Subject throws with unaffected hand and catches with affected hand. He can rather precisely throw it to the place where his affected hand is, obviating eye-hand coordination. Subtasks: 1 throw, 1 catch. Total number: 2
- (Ball Back) The subject could not predict the coordinates of the point where he would have to bring his affected hand to catch the ball, thus necessitating eye-hand coordination. Subtasks: 1 throw, 1 catch, 1 eye-hand coordination. Total number: 3
- (TWO) As the subject had considerable problems extending the index finger this was counted as a separate subtask. This problem was much less pronounced for any other finger. Subtasks: 1 extension, 2 flexions, 1 translation. Total number: 4
- (TWOPLUS) Subtasks: 1 extension, 2 flexions, 1 thumb touch, translation. Total number 5
- (THREE) Subtasks: 1 extension, 3 flexions, 1 translation. Total number: 5
- (FOUR) Subtasks: 1 extension, 4 flexions, 1 translation. Total number: 6
- (FOURPLUS) Subtasks: 1 extension, 4 flexions, 1 thumb touch, 1 translation. Total number: 7
- (WAFERS10) Subtasks: 1 extension, 4 flexions, 2 translations (to type the numerals). Total number: 7
- (Fox) Since the subject typed with four fingers on the left and right side, it can be argued every flexion on the left side had to be integrated with the motion and rhythm of the right hand, so that a separate subtask can be assigned to each flexion: the flexion integration. Subtasks: 1 extension, 4 flexions, 4 integrations. Total number: 9.

The time constants have been plotted versus the number of subtasks in Figure ApII–2. The subtasks are clearly not identical and in Figure ApII–2 only their number is used and not their nature. Using an operational definition we have called the number of subtasks the complexity c of an exercise. This is not a unique identifier, some tasks are distinct but have the same number of subtasks, hence the same complexity. The idea that a more complex task takes more time to learn was plausible and for lack of better insight a linear relationship was expected.

We have fitted the data of Figure ApII–2 with a best-fitting straight line, which is also plotted. The expression we found for this line is:

$$\tau(c) = 35.5 + 29.3c \qquad\qquad (4)$$

from which we conclude that every subtask adds 29 days to the time constants.

Considerable doubt exists about the validity of the subtask analysis. For example the time constant for TWOPLUS (182 days) is smaller than for TWO (197 days), although the former requires an extra thumb touch to the spacebar. A similar paradox exist between FOUR and FOURPLUS, where the extra thumb touch reduces the time constant from 202 to 190 days. It might be that the extra touch

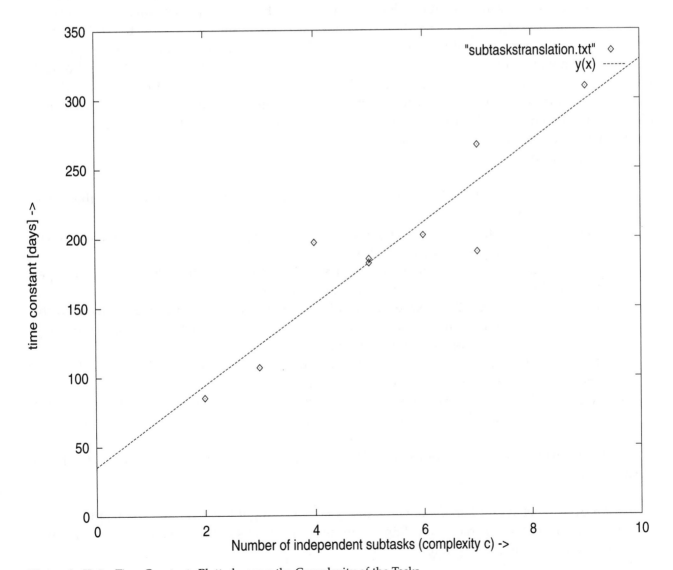

Figure ApII–2   Time Constants Plotted versus the Complexity of the Tasks

is not a hand movement but rather a clockwise flick of the forearm, while the hands stays rigid. It has been observed that the unaffected hand of the subject performed an associate movement in which the right forearm makes a fast counterclockwise flick, which helped the subject maintain balance. It is speculated that this associated movement helped the affected left hand to such an extent that a negative time contribution was achieved in both exercises. Similar reinforcements have been suggested by Brunnstrom [11], though without documented results.

After 120 days of exercising, the subject changed the endurance exercise from the 10 minutes on the exercise bike to a one-hour walk in the neighborhood. He kept on performing all exercises once per day. It was observed that his performance deteriorated in all exercises. The reason for this deterioration was not clear. He was checked for new brain damage, which apparently had not occurred. In order to reverse the deterioration, the subject changed his regimen from doing every exercise once per day to executing every exercise three times per day. He kept on walking as an endurance exercise. This extra effort paid off; he was able to stem his deterioration, and after about three months he began so see a sustained improvement again. At day 260, it was speculated that the change in endurance exercise had provoked the deterioration, and the subject resumed his bike exercises for endurance. The results were dramatic; in less than a week, he had registered improvement in all exercises of a magnitude of 20 to 30 percent, as compared to a daily improvements of 0.3 to 1.0 percent per day due to the normal repetition in the exercises. The large influence of this effect was probably due to the removal of muscle stiffness as it occurred on the exercises bike, but not during the walking, since then the arm is only dangling alongside the body. The subject felt much less pain during the day in the affected side after he resumed the bike exercises than during the period in which he did the walking. From day 229 to 240 all exercises were suspended. When they were resumed again, a large deterioration (30 to 50 percent) was observed in all exercises.

Six regimens of exercise can be discerned

1. Regimen A (day 1–120). All exercise are performed once per day; for endurance, the subject used the exercise bike.
2. Regimen B (day 120–160). As in regimen A, but walking for endurance instead of exercise biking. The subject is not aware of his deterioration.
3. Regimen C (day 160–220). Subject becomes aware of deterioration. All exercises are performed three times per day, still walking for endurance.
4. Regimen D (day 230–240). No exercises at all. The subject deteriorates 28 percent in this exercise and performs on day 240 as on day 75 (in other words, he lost the effect of 165 days of exercising by not exercising for 10 days).
5. Regimen E (day 240–253). Same as regimen C (three performances per day and walking for endurance). Downwards trend of regimen C continues.
6. Regimen F (day 253–365). Three performances per day and exercise bike for endurance. Rapid improvement during first week of regimen F.

In Figure ApII–3, the results of exercise FOUR are presented by way of example. This figure illustrates several points:

• An overall behavior of an exponential decay curve (straight line in a logarithmic plot).
• Change from bike exercise to walking exercise leads to considerable deterioration of the performance, starting at day 120.

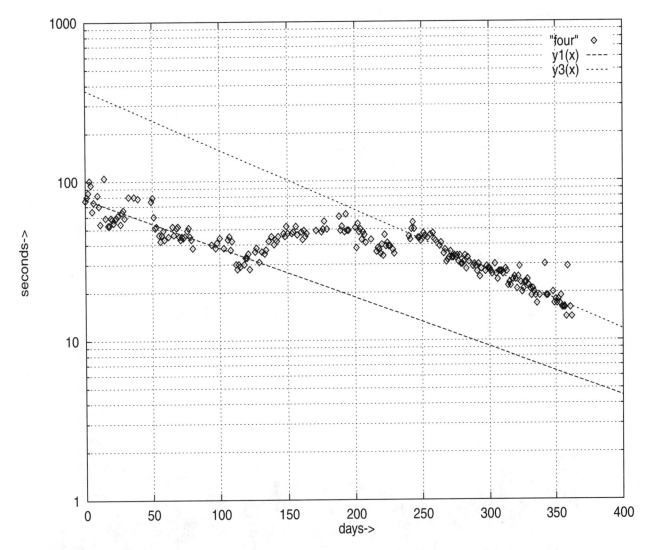

Figure ApII–3 Performance in Exercise FOUR. (This performance shows many aspects of the recovery.)

- Change from one execution of an exercise to three executions per day reversed the deterioration. This occurred during day 170–229.
- Keeping all exercises (including the endurance exercise) constant resulted in a continuation of the straight line in the logarithmic plot.
- Suspension of exercises resulted in large deterioration (days 229–245).
- The slope in the area where the subject performed the exercise once per day, while also exercise biking (-0.0071), indicated with function $y_1(x)$, is close to the slope in the area where the exercises were performed three times per day, while also biking (-0.0087), indicated by function $y_3(x)$. This suggests that the extra two performances contributed relatively little over just the first performance.

THE OVERALL PERSPECTIVE

In Figure ApII–4, the results of all measurements for the duration of one year is given in a log-line plot. Although this figure is very cluttered and individual curves cannot easily be identified, the general appearance is clear. There is continued recovery as long as there have been exercises. There is no observation of leveling off to a plateau.

RESULTS

The performance of a stroke patient has been quantified in exercises measuring the speed in finishing a task, as well as exercises measuring the quality of the performance.

No leveling-off to a plateau was observed in any exercise.

The performances have been identified as exponential decay functions.

Every exercise had its own recovery rate time constant.

The complexity of exercises had been operationally defined as the number of subtasks of an exercise. The time constant of an exercise was found to be linearly proportional to its complexity.

The influence of vigorous arm exercise on an exercise bike with hand-pedals, on the hand recovery process has been established, and has been found to be very large.

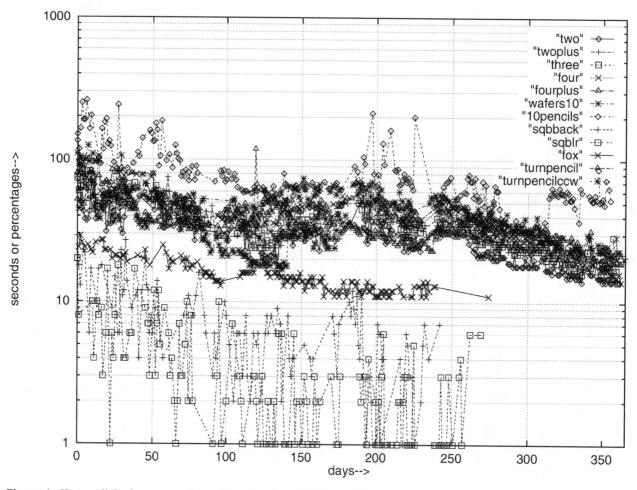

Figure ApII–4   All Performances Shown Together for a Full Year of Exercising

ACKNOWLEDGMENTS

The author is indebted for the many hours of fruitful discussions to Professor Catherine A. Trombly, Sc.D., OTR/L, who teaches Occupational Therapy at the Sargent College for Health and Rehabilitation Sciences at Boston University, and to Dr. Serge H. Roy, Sc.D. PT, staff therapist at the Neuromuscular Research Center in the College of Engineering at Boston University.

CONCLUSIONS

In a therapeutic setting, more emphasis should be placed on quantitative determination of the performance, as a sense of real achievement of recovery is of the greatest importance to a patient.

The design of a series of exercises, which are repeatable and easily measurable, deserves serious consideration from members of the therapeutic community.

Since the time constants are large (hundreds of days) it is important that patients continue their exercises for a long time, longer than conventional insurance programs currently allow in their benefits packages. So patients should continue exercising at home, for instance by using exercise workbooks.

References

1. Duncan, P.W., Goldstein, L.B., Horner, R.D., Landsman, P.B., Samsa, G.P., & Matchar, D.B. (1994). Similar motor recovery of upper and lower extremities after stroke. *Stroke*, 25(6), 1181–1188.

2. Jorgensen, H.S., Nakayama, H., Raaschou, H.O., Vive-Larsen, J., Stoier, M., & Olsen, T.S. (1955). Outcome and time course of recovery in stroke, part I: Outcome. The Copenhagen stroke study. *Arch. Phys. Med Rehabil*, 76, 399–405.

3. Partridge, C.J., & Edwards, S. (1988). Recovery curves as basis for evaluation. *Physiotherapy*, 74(3), 141–143.

4. Partridge, C.J. (1992). Describing patterns of recovery as a basis for evaluating progress. *International Journal on Technology Assessment in Health Care*, 8(1), 55–61.

5. Parker, V.M., Wade, T.D., & Langton Hewer, R. (1986). Loss of arm function after stroke, measurement frequency and recovery. *Int. Rehabil.Med*, 8, 69–73.

6. Dombovy, M.L., & Bach-y-Rita, P. (1988). Clinical observations on recovery from stroke. *Advances in Neurology*, 47, Functional recovery in neurological disease. New York: Raven Press.

7. Duncan, P.W., Goldstein, L.B., Matchar, D., Divine, G.W., & Feussner J. (1992). Measurement of motor recovery after stroke. *Stroke*, 23(8), 1084–1089.

8. Freund, H.J. (1996). Remapping the brain. *Science*, 272, 1754.

9. Nudo, R.J., Wise, B.M., SiFuentes, F., & Milliken, G.W. (1996). Neural substrates for the effects of rehabilitative training on motor recovery after ischemic infarct. *Science*, 272, 1791–1794.

10. Nudo, R.J., Milliken, G.W., Jenkins, W. M., & Merzenich, M.M. (1966) Use dependent alterations of movement representations in primary motor cortex on adult squirrel monkeys. *J. NeuroScience*, 16(2), 785–809.

11. Brunnstrom, S. (1970). *Movement Therapy in Hemiplegia*. New York: Harper & Row.

Appendix III

Keyboard Layout and Finger Usage

In Figure ApIII–1 you will find a diagram of which finger goes with which key in typing exercises. You can use this diagram with the typing exercises in Chapters 24 through 33.

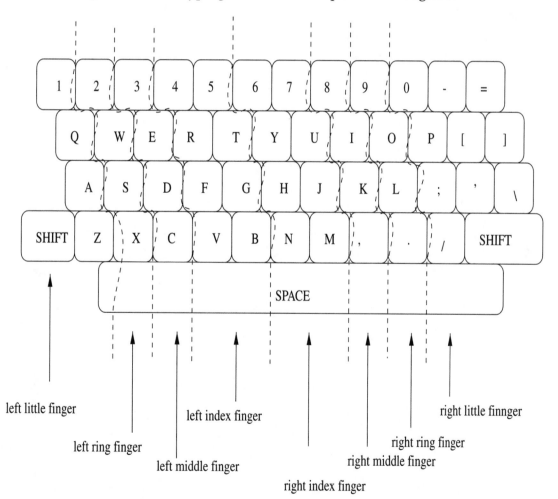

Figure ApIII–1   Diagram Finger Usage in Typing Exercises

Appendix IV

Determining Averages and Time Constants

AVERAGES

In this book you measure your own performance (in most exercises, three times in a row) and calculate and plot the average in graphs.

To determine the average of three numbers you add the three numbers and divide the result by 3. Let us imagine that you did an exercise three times, and that you finished the exercise in 33, 37, and 39 seconds. To find the average, add the three numbers and divide the result by 3:

Adding the three numbers: 33 + 37 + 39 = 109

Divide the result by three: 109/3 = 36 1/3 = 36.33

Round off to the nearest whole number: 36

A TRICK TO MAKE YOUR LIFE EASIER

If you want a simple, quick way of doing the calculation, here is a little trick. Instead of adding up the three numbers and dividing by 3, determine which number is the smallest and what the difference is between the smallest number and the other two numbers. Then add up those differences, divide that result by 3, and add this result to the smallest number. In the following example of this method, we use the same numbers as in the previous example (33, 37, and 39).

The smallest number is 33. The differences between 33 and the other two numbers are:

for 37: 37 − 33 = 4
for 39: 39 − 33 = 6

Add the 4 and the 6 together, divide the result by 3: 4 + 6 = 10; 10/3 = 3 1/3. Add this to the smallest number: 33 + 3 1/3 = 36 1/3.

As you will see, you get the same result as before. This method is easier, and you will probably be able to do it in your head if the part of your brain that has been damaged does not involve calculation (mostly, the left side of the brain). Doing the calculation in your head also activates the brain.

TIME CONSTANTS

You can determine the time constants of any particular exercise in the logarithmic plots. I suggest that you determine the time constant for each exercise after four months of exercising. It is a good idea to keep on exercising for a period of time equal to two times the time constant of each exercise. Since all exercises are different, they all have different time constants, so you will have to do some exercises longer than others.

The determination of a time constant consists of two steps.

1. First, determine what the best straight line is through the points of the plot. (The best straight line is the line that has the smallest total distance to all points.) Since there are many points, there is no simple answer to this problem. There are two ways of finding the best straight line:

   (a) By using a computer program. In order to find the best straight line you can use Mathematica[1] software. This calculates the total distance of all points to an arbitrary straight line and then determines which straight line has the smallest total distance to all points. This is an exact method. If you use Mathematica, store the results of your performance in a file named EXERCISE.DAT (where EXERCISE could be any exercise name; e.g., QW or THREE or Philosopher). Include in the file two numbers for everyday. The first number is the day number, the second number is the performance.

   This routine is called BFCALC, after "best fit calculation." First you read in the file numbers, then the subroutine. It will automatically calculate the time constant, the slope, and the point where the straight line crosses the vertical axis. When using Mathematica, at the prompt, type in the command to read the file, and load the subroutine. To read the file type:

   In[1]=p=ReadList["EXERCISE.DAT",{Number,Number}]

   Notice the two capital letters in **ReadList**, as well as those in **Number,Number** and the quotes around the filename **EXERCISE.DAT**. Also notice the square brackets—[]—and the curly braces—{ }. After the new Mathematica prompt, type:

   In[2] = << BFCALC

   This is two left-pointing arrows followed by the subroutine. You may have to find out how to get the left-pointing arrows. On some keyboards, there are special keys for them; on others, you have to use the SHIFT key and the comma or the period key.

   Mathematica will now print "timeconstant," "slope," and "vertical intercept," and will give the numbers. The following is a subroutine:

```
pt = Transpose[p]
pt[[2]] = Log[pt[[2]]]
fitmatrix11 = 2 pt[[1]]. pt[[1]]
n = Dimensions[pt[[1]]][[1]]
unitvector = Table [1,i,n]
fitmatrix12 = 2 pt[[1]] .unitvector
fitmatrix21 = fitmatrix12
fitmatrix22 = 2 n
fitmatrix = {fitmatrix11, fitmatrix12, fitmatrix21, fitmatrix22}
```

```
MatrixForm[fitmatrix]
rightside = {2 pt[[1]]. pt[[2]], 2 pt[[2]]. unitvector}
solution = Inverse[fitmatrix]. rightside
intercept = N[solution[[2]]]
slope = N[solution[[1]]]
timeconstant = -1/slope
Print["timeconstant=", timeconstant]
Print["intercept=", intercept]
```

(b) The second method gives an approximate result that in most cases will be surprisingly accurate and will differ only a little from the result of the Mathematica method. In this method, you guess what the best straight line is using your eyes and your best judgment. Scientists call this method "eyeballing." Place a clear plastic ruler on the plot and move it around a little bit so that a single line drawn along the ruler through this cloud of points will be, in your judgment, the best straight line through all these points.

2. Once you have found the best straight line, you can determine the time constant. You will notice that your best straight line intersects all horizontal lines. Now find where the best straight line intersects two horizontal lines that are a separated by a factor of 2 (for instance, the lines for 10 and 20, or for 50 and 100, or for 100 and 200).

Let us assume that you use the lines for 50 and 100. (Any set of two lines that are separated by a factor of 2 will give the same result.) Mark the point where your best straight line intersects the line for 50 with a cross (X). Mark the point where your best straight line intersects the line for 100 with a small circle (o). With the ruler, draw vertical lines through the cross and the circle. Now determine how many days there are between the two vertical lines. Multiply that number of days by 1.4; the result is the time constant of this exercise.

For instance, let us assume that the vertical line through the circle intersects the time axis at day 12, and the vertical line through the cross at day 168, the number of days between the vertical lines, is 168 – 12 = 156. In that case, the time constant of that exercise is 156 x 1.4 = 218.4 days.

---

[1]Mathematica is a trademark belonging to Wolfram Research, Inc.

Never forget who your friends are
Or who your family is
When they are still alive
The dead live forever
The living are often forgotten
and are taken for granted.
I will never forget that Jan's brother came
when Jan was in the hospital with a stroke.
Leo came and listened to my endless babble,
stricken with fear,
and desperate himself.
Jan lifted his arm for him in the hospital,
to wave goodbye to him, his heavy paralyzed arm.
We will remember with great love that his sister-in-law
Yvonne came to help him exercise and learn to relax
and instilled a bit of trust in ourselves.
How our neighbors helped so much,
we became friends for life.
How Jan's parents called every week for two years in a row,
how all our friends helped.
When we brought Jan home from the hospital, we knew
that all those people that cared and helped so much,
in reality brought him home.

—Else

Index